*Flying
Without Wings*

ARNOLD R. BEISSER

Flying Without Wings

Personal Reflections on Loss, Disability, and Healing

Foreword by Hugh Prather and Gerald Jampolsky, M.D.

BANTAM BOOKS
NEW YORK · TORONTO · LONDON · SYDNEY · AUCKLAND

This edition contains the complete text
of the original hardcover edition.
NOT ONE WORD HAS BEEN OMITTED.

FLYING WITHOUT WINGS
A Bantam Book / published by arrangement with
Doubleday

PRINTING HISTORY
Doubleday edition published January 1989
Bantam edition / March 1990

Library of Congress Cataloging-in-Publication Data

Beisser, Arnold R.
  Flying without wings : personal reflections on being disabled ;
foreword by Hugh Prather and Gerald Jampolsky. — Bantam ed.
      p.   cm.
  Reprint. Originally published: New York : Doubleday, 1989.
  ISBN: 978-0-553-34868-2
  1. Beisser, Arnold R.—Health.   2. Psychiatrists—California—
Biography.   3. Paralytics—California—Biography.   I. Title.
RC438.6.B45A3   1990
616.89'0092—dc20
[B]   89-15116
                                                        CIP

Published simultaneously in the United States and Canada

Bantam Books are published by Bantam Books, a division of Bantam
Doubleday Dell Publishing Group, Inc. Its trademark, consisting of the
words "Bantam Books" and the portrayal of a rooster, is Registered
in U.S. Patent and Trademark Office and in other countries. Marca
Registrada. Bantam Books, 666 Fifth Avenue, New York, New York 10103.

PRINTED IN THE UNITED STATES OF AMERICA

13

To Mae Beisser Elkins

Acknowledgments

The Phillips Foundation
Jack and Helen Levin
The Suicide Prevention Center
Rita Beisser
Dalia Blitzer
Gerta Prosser

Foreword

Hugh Prather and Gerald Jampolsky, M.D.

DOWN THROUGH the ages, from a hundred different cultures, from a thousand different teachings, have come the concepts of surrender and acceptance, of focus and commitment, of humor and perspective, of internal discipline or living in the present, and of forgiveness or complete kindness. But it has often been assumed that although this perennial wisdom remains the same, it is really a mental plaything for the comfortably situated and is partially, if not wholly, impractical for those who struggle and suffer and even for those whose lives contain a common measure of hardship.

In our work with the bereaved, the catastrophically ill, and others in crisis, we have seen that, on the contrary, the more desperately these concepts are needed and the more wholeheartedly they are turned to, the more enormous is their potential for delivering a growing sense of peace and even glimpses of a higher reality. However, both of us are able-bodied, and although we have had our share of pain, we are perceived by others as having a good lot in life and thus can safely speak of love and joy, having essentially no real cause for any other emotions. It is therefore with gratitude that we have watched Arnold Beisser revise this manuscript and with each draft recount more of the personal circumstances that give this book its unique power. The editor at Doubleday who accepted it said, "This is a Godsend for the disabled," and to us it is equally a supreme gift to the able-bodied, becuase it so clearly shows the application of fundamental truth under conditions that before have been considered preclusive.

Arnie would never describe himself as enlightened or even more advanced than others. But when a man who suddenly finds himself a quadriplegic in an iron lung can come to say, "My life is enough," who can fail to listen? Arnie would not claim to have done any more than try hard and make a few modest gains. And yet this is the key to progress. His mental wholeness was gained the way any individual must attain it: by taking, in great humility, one small step at a time.

The person who makes the greatest progress is the one who has stopped waiting for an all-encompassing breakthrough and has settled for a little gain each day. Humans never quite manage to adhere perfectly to the schedule they have set for their own inner improvement. Therefore, individuals who are truly sincere must simply surrender *some,* or meditate *some,* or serve others *some,* or hold to an honest thought *some.* And they must do it today.

As anyone can attest who has done in-depth counseling with a large variety of people, the heart of any individual contains ample stores of good, simple wisdom. It's not that we don't already know enough to begin living lives of gentleness and peace, but we all have a little picture of how things must look before we can begin. There are several conditions that are not quite right. First we will straighten these out and then we will begin being the kind of person we deeply long to be. But, of course, there is no end to what needs setting right, and as soon as one problem is behind us another takes its place.

Of this you can be sure. Enough will happen today to make you miserable. Enough will happen today to justify waiting a little longer. Surely enough happened in Arnold Beisser's life. The only difference is that he chose not to wait.

There is no better life than the one you have. There is no better time than now. The only day in which you can begin your journey into the light of your own heart is today, because it will never stop being today. Sooner or later an instant must come in which you take up the burdens of your life and go forth. And this is what Arnold

Beisser shows is a present possibility for any individual, no matter what his or her circumstances.

Yet once this journey into the holy instant is begun, nothing but the journey itself can be anticipated as a reward. There may be other pleasant fallouts, but they cannot be counted on. Arnold Beisser's body never got substantially better and how deeply are we all blessed that it did not. In our new age preoccupation with so-called higher laws, with religious invocations and metaphysical manipulations, when now the mind can supposedly shape the course of events to "whatever you want badly enough," it is often overlooked that Jesus' life did not go well. Nor did the lives of so many other masters the world has been touched and blessed by. Jesus did not have the respect of the colleagues in his chosen profession. He did not achieve his earning potential. His friends did not remain loyal. His students did not keep the faith. He did not die a peaceful death surrounded by admirers. His teaching did not remain unperverted. And two thousand years later everything he represented is still being cruelly misinterpreted and misused. In short, at the end of his life he had nothing to show for his time, nothing, that is, that the world holds dear. And yet he achieved all.

Within these pages is a modern parallel, another chance at sanity. Here is a man who lived a real life and yet reached for love's vision. Here is one whom worldly circumstances did not treat fairly and yet who chose to forgive everything and turned to bless the world as best he could. The lesson is clear. Anyone can bless. Therefore anyone can have the peace of heart, the lightness of giving, and the gentle and deep reward that Arnold Beisser has increasingly experienced.

HUGH: Both of us have been deeply affected by our contact with Arnie's powerful and very pure gentleness. How this book came into print is one small example. For many years Jerry related instances to me of Arnie's profound inner growth in the face of hardships so extreme that they were, to me, unimaginable. In 1986, Jerry told me that Arnie had completed a manuscript about his life, and at his suggestion I phoned him to talk about the book. He sent it to me, and after looking it over I offered to submit it to the editor who was handling Gayle and me at that time.

A month or so after mailing it, I asked about the status of the manuscript and was told it had not yet been read. I waited another month, inquired again, and was told the same. In short, this pattern continued for about six months, at which time I was informed that it had been rejected but could not be returned because it had been misplaced. I kept Arnie apprised of all this. After repeated follow-up inquiries (because I was not really sure the manuscript had even been read), I finally had to tell Arnie that I could not get his book published, and furthermore, I could not even get it back.

It is just another indication of the strength of Arnie's gentleness that in 1988 when I offered to submit his second draft to a new editor that he not only agreed, but when I reminded him of what had happened the last time, he had so thoroughly put it from his mind that at first he did not even recall the series of mishaps. As you read this book, you will feel within him this powerful absence of grievances as he recounts events, any one of which would seem sufficient provocation for a lifetime of bitterness. In my opinion, it is the purity of the mind behind it, so remarkably clean of all anger and attack, that causes this book to be deeply healing. Arnold Beisser's account emblazons the heart with one liberating truth: Nothing in this world, nothing in another's behavior, or even in one's own physical makeup or functioning, can poison one's life. Only the mind can blot out the peace of the heart and infect a life with darkness, and only the mind can release the heart to grandeur.

It is crucial to understand that when this man began his first tentative efforts, he was neither a genius nor a saint. Nor was he in possession of some extraordinary philosophy. He had, in fact, only one remaining strength: the willingness to try. And what he accomplished in a lifetime so far outweighs the usual professional, physical, or monetary accomplishment that comparisons are impossible. Nothing can be weighed in the balance of love. And it is into this realm of reality that Arnold Beisser has begun to walk, and gently leads us all.

JERRY: I have known Arnie for forty-two years. We met as first-year medical students at Stanford Medical School, where we became roommates, and have remained close friends since that time. What immediately impressed me and always has about Arnie is his deep sense of integrity and sincerity, a consistently caring attitude toward others, a smile and sense of humor that I like to bathe in, and a strong inner knowledge that nothing of true value is impossible.

Arnie worked hard at medical school, but sports were his first love. It was beautiful to watch him play tennis, with his sense of single-minded concentration, strength, fair play, and a grace that I had never witnessed before. On occasions he would go out on the court and "toy around" with me. By this I mean he would give me the great advantage in terms of points and would proceed to wipe me out, six–love, six–love!

I don't remember anybody not loving Arnie. He was elected president of our medical school class, and was and is one of the few people I know who simply never attracts enemies. Arnie not only has been a warm and trusted friend, but he has taught me that we each have within us a potential, a spirit, a vision that does not perceive limits because it does not include any. I feel so privileged to have experienced such a long and enduring friendship, and I am delighted that we have been so free along the way to openly acknowledge our respect and love for each other. Our families have been intertwined and the person to whom this book is dedicated, Arnie's mother, has always had a very special place in my heart.

When I think of Arnie, I think of his joy. Many are the times we have happily reminisced about medical school. Without his sense of humor I don't believe he would have made it, and his chapter on humor is a classic. Reading *Flying Without Wings* reminds me of a letter I received some years ago from a fifteen-year-old quadraplegic boy who had seen me on a television special about our center. He wrote: "I really believe in what you guys are doing. You see, I don't think there is any such thing as handicapped bodies: I think there are only handicapped minds."

There were many times when I would visit Arnie after he came down with polio that I wondered if I would ever see him again. His body was so withered that I felt the slightest illness would cause his death. But Arnie has an unstoppable spirit that refuses to be defeated.

By far the most overwhelming experience I had with Arnie was the day I received a letter from him about a dramatic change in his work. Arnie's situation at that time was that he had worked very hard and had made Metropolitan State Hospital in Southern California into one of the finest teaching hospitals in the country. He and Rita were quite comfortable there. They had a house, many aids to help Arnie, and things seemed to be going so well for both of them. But Arnie stated in his letter that he was resigning because he needed a new challenge! He had decided to take the position of Director of the Center for Training in Community Psychiatry for Southern California.

I cried on reading this letter. Here he had accomplished so much more than someone in his condition could ever expect to, and yet he was not content to rest on his laurels. Helping people to remove the blocks to the realization that no internal gain is impossible has become a major part of my work at the Center for Attitudinal Healing and Arnold Beisser was one of the first and most influential teachers in my learning the validity of this concept.

I cannot pretend to be objective about *Flying Without Wings*. Yet, in the deepest part of my heart I believe this book will be of tremendous help to all of us who have emotional and physical challenges. Arnie writes with a clarity beyond words about his own "inside conversations," which put a new light on the perceptions of a patient who has become quadriplegic. Arnie is an usher with a very bright flashlight into this inner world, and he explores it with wisdom and humor. Yet, in the fullest sense, Arnie *demonstrates* a "positive state of health." The wholeness of life can be experienced by meeting challenges with limitless spirit and love, which are inherent in each of our minds and hearts. And this my old friend and teacher has done.

Contents

1

Time

As if you could kill time without injuring eternity.

—Henry David Thoreau

ALL THAT I HAVE in life is a little time. Perhaps that is all anyone ever has. I am aware that time is very precious and not too much is left.

When I was a child, if my mother said that I had an hour to play it seemed like a lifetime. The possibilities within that time were limitless. I had very little past, and the future seemed entirely open. Time moved very slowly.

Perhaps from a need to lay out some benchmarks, I wrote a life plan when I was ten. Although I forgot all about the plan, my mother did not, and years later she resurrected it, and to my great embarrassment proudly showed it to her friends.

The first item said: Win national tennis championship by age twenty-three. (I had looked up the ages of all national tennis champions and discovered this was the average.) The second item: Obtain a doctorate by age twenty-seven. (I do not know why I selected twenty-seven, except that it seemed about as young as was dignified for one to be a doctor.) The third item was get married and settle down by age thirty.

The first two items presented few complications. I won my national tennis championship at twenty-four, and completed medical school at twenty-three, well ahead of schedule. These and other experiences were providing me with a respectable past. As I was busily engaged in work and play, my personal sense of time had quickened.

The year was 1950, and President Truman sent the U.S. armed forces to fight in Korea. As a Navy reserve officer, I was ordered to report. At my first station I was examined, pronounced physically fit, and given new orders for duty. But en route I developed a fever and entered a nearby naval hospital. There was an unexpected change of plans in my childhood agenda, and there began a future life for which I was totally unprepared. Without warning, my body had failed me. In a few hours I was transformed from a doctor to a patient, from an athlete to a cripple. Polio ravaged me so that I could not move. I could not stand, walk, sit, eat, drink, or even breathe by myself.

When I first got sick, I could move nothing below my head and I even had some paralysis of my face. For the entire first year and a half, I lay flat on my back in an iron lung. I was hospitalized for three years and there was some very gradual improvement, but hardly enough to be noticed.

The person I had known myself to be was quite suddenly trapped in an alien body—one which did not perform automatically on command, or indeed even perform at all.

As a consequence, I came to know time in a quite different way. I would ask a nurse what time it was. She would answer, "One o'clock." I would then wait and wait and wait. After what seemed two or three hours, I would ask again. Her answer might be: "Three minutes after one." I was sure it was a trick, some practical joke designed to torment me. I knew what an hour was like, and the difference between a couple of hours and a couple of minutes. Similar episodes were repeated over and over with different people at every hour of the day and night. Minutes and seconds seemed endless.

The mass that I had called my body had changed, and time had changed with it. I learned firsthand about relative qualities of time and space. Although I hardly interpreted the subject in such a lofty mode, I had a little peek into what Einstein had described. Without motion, time seemed to have slowed so considerably that it almost stopped.

The smooth flow from past to present to future had ceased. Without familiar sources of pleasure and meaning, there was no future. Those things I had been moving toward were gone; they had simply disappeared. The movement of time was blocked, making the present interminable, lifeless, and dead.

The past, however, was a different story. I spent my time reviewing it as a moment of glory, detailing its pleasures, and even its failures. The past had expanded as the future had closed.

I began to understand that the kind of time I was now living by was dramatically different from my past experience of time duration. I had told time, subjectively, before, by moving through space and utilizing the benchmarks of accomplishments. Now, as I lay helpless, completely passive, my own time had stopped moving. The tedium this produced was agonizing, broken only by my efforts to put into thoughts and words what was happening to me.

I wondered what the limits were to the experience of time's passing. If time slows almost to a stop when one is inactive and uninvolved, could it also accelerate to infinity if one were fully absorbed? Could I ever reach it? And what kind of ecstasy might that state be?

I had caught a glimpse of what it could be like on a few memorable occasions. There was a day many years ago when I was playing in a tennis tournament against a highly ranked player who ordinarily would have beaten me easily. This day, without preparation, all struggle and effort began to disappear. In its place there emerged a wonderful feeling of calm, ease, and fluidity. I moved about the court without strain, seemingly part of some greater unity. All of my activity, and that of my opponent, seemed like parts of one unified whole, and I seemed to get to the place where the ball was arriving without trying. My shots landed in my opponent's court exactly where I directed them. Winning or losing was unimportant. In this incredible experience I was fully absorbed into the moment. I did not try to win, and although to the amazement of onlookers I won handily, I did not care. All I cared about was the fullness of the present, and there was nothing else. I do not know how I got into that state, nor do I know how it passed from me.

There were other times. I recall once on a basketball court when I and all of the players on both teams became part of a miraculous ballet, choreographed to perfection. When I took a shot, there was no question the ball was destined to go through the hoop.

As I lay motionless, I thought about these moments of perfection and harmony. I felt discouraged, for they all involved intense physical activity. Now I was immobilized, and it seemed unlikely that the ingredients for similar experiences would ever again be present.

My physical world had shrunk to the small room that contained my iron lung. My field of vision was limited to the ceiling and what was reflected in the mirror on my iron lung. In the evening, when the world grew darker, my world shrank further. I could no longer see the pattern on the ceiling, and the reflection in the mirror was dim. Not until two years later, in my fourth hospital, could I turn my head to the side enough to look down a corridor outside my room.

One evening, lying there alone, feeling particularly hopeless and bored, I looked down the corridor wishing for, perhaps expecting, someone or something. But I saw only the darkened hallway with a few doors opening onto it. There was no activity, and there were no people to be seen. My despair mounted, and I felt as though I could no longer stand it. Then, slowly, I began to look at the corridor differently, and I began to see variations, shades of gray and darkness, shadows and light. The doorways opening onto the corridor formed subtle geometric patterns according to the different ways the doors were ajar. I began to look carefully and wonder at this scene that only a few moments before had depressed me so. It now seemed startlingly beautiful. My perception had shifted, my eyes miraculously refreshed. This experience was full and whole. I looked down the hallway for a very long time. I think that at last I probably fell asleep, but I am not sure.

I do not know how that perception arrived, or why it left, but from then on I understood that what I sought was possible. My task now was to discover how to change from the one state to the other.

I had to look for that magic element. I knew now that it did not reveal itself in the hands of the clock, but its secret was somewhere *between* the ticks of the clock. It is a place far more immediate than the past, and far more certain than the future.

But I was not ready to understand meanings. Other things were more urgent. It looked like I was going to survive. But what kind of life could it be? It would be a living death unless I could find some way of getting some satisfaction out of it. "You only know what you know" is an obvious saying, but a profound one. The only satisfactions I could comprehend were those I had known before, such as playing sports or spending time with women. But those pleasures now seemed unattainable, for they depended on being as I was before. That is the dilemma for everyone after losing something or someone that is important. "You only know what you know."

Athletics had been the most important single thing in my life. I worked and I went to school, but always the reward for doing these "worthwhile" things was that I could then go out and play basketball or tennis or some other sport. Sports were the consuming interest of my life.

Some of my thoughts about sports were very bizarre. But then, I was leading a new life, and I suppose I could not be expected to live it well immediately. At the naval hospital the first year, I sometimes had heard conversations about table tennis among the doctors and nurses. A plan began to develop in my mind, based on past experience.

I had been quite a good table tennis player. In fact, I had often played with various handicaps for money. For example, sometimes I sat in a chair and/or used a makeshift paddle, such as a book.

I began to conceive of my disability as similar to those handicaps I had taken on voluntarily to equalize the competition. If I could stay out of the respirator for half an hour, I could perhaps be propped in a wheelchair, and if I could move my arm just a little, I could play. I thought I could still show my skill, and what a wonderful challenge it could be! The potential pleasure of beating my opponent with the challenge of the ultimate handicap occupied me for days. Only the passage of time, and with it the realization of the true extent of my paralysis, made this fantasy gradually disappear.

Now that I was no longer able to participate in any

sport, or for that matter to have any physical expression of my body, I had an enormous amount of pent-up energy with which to deal. At first I had mainly my past in sports to remember, and I reviewed every match, every game, every play in meticulous detail. But then I began to find a new expression for my interest in sports. I became a real sports fan for the first time. Before, I had been bored by the performances of others. Now, however, I began to savor the role that was available to me—that of a spectator.

Someone brought me a radio within a few weeks after I became ill, and later another friend brought a small television set. (In 1950 television sets were not readily available in hospitals.) Looking through the iron lung mirror at a television set is disorienting at first, because everything is backwards. Left-handed baseball pitchers were right-handed, and players ran around the bases the wrong way. But I watched and listened hungrily. This became my way of filling the emptiness of time.

Something else happened. Without realizing it I was beginning to view my disability as a competitive sport, and to translate that view into the urgent business at hand.

Once again I used achievement to tell time. My first task was to attain my maximum level of rehabilitation—to become as close to my former self as possible. I did not think to question whether this was a worthwhile goal.

I constructed a new timetable based on my progress to that point. If I could breathe outside the iron lung for five minutes after a month, I reasoned that I should be able to stay out an hour after a year. If I could accelerate that pace, I could begin thinking about doing other things—sitting up, going places, seeing friends. With these possibilities, the future opened a little, and the importance of the past began to recede; with these changes, the pace of time in the present quickened once again.

As with my pre-polio timetable, I wanted to go faster and faster—to exceed the timetable I had planned. I competed with time as though it was my opponent.

My self-esteem was at a very low ebb, and I had much to catch up with, and much that was unfinished. I began my tasks once again as though the future was endless and my goal was to beat time and get past certain benchmarks.

I began to set other goals too, ones that had to do with achieving a profession, going to work, developing relationships, and writing—perhaps. I thought achievements could make me feel worthwhile again and give me self-respect.

But my search was based on a misunderstanding of time. The major transition needed was from seeing life as competition to experiencing it much more simply and directly for what it was.

As I now think about those timetables for myself, I am reminded of a cartoon I once saw in *The New Yorker:* two weary men were talking in a bar, and one said to the other, ". . . and then you're too old to think about becoming the youngest anything." But I was not yet ready to realize that time was not for a race, and that I did not have an opponent other than myself to beat.

Most of the things that I tried to do involved leaving other parts of myself behind. I was trying to be exactly as I was before. But that was trying to recapture what was only a memory. My more important task was to integrate my past with things in my present: somehow to put together the many torn fragments of my life.

When I was fully absorbed with what I was doing, time moved so quickly that I was nowhere but in the present. There was then no longer anything to seek, and I was no longer in a race. I had moments when I would experience that limitless present—what the ancient wisdom had called the "holy instant," when there was no time and there were no divisions, and when I was fully manifest.

Such revelations occurred under many circumstances: sometimes when an experience was particularly moving, as with another person; sometimes when I was in awe of great beauty or grotesqueness; sometimes when some mysterious process would open my perceptions so that I could see in a new way. But perhaps the most important of these instances was when the slender thread that kept me alive was threatened, and I became aware with full force that my life was temporal, and that it could be over at any moment. My survival was so precarious that it could be threatened at any moment. For example, since I could not cough, sneeze, or blow my nose, a common cold was life-threatening. Recognizing the preciousness of this opportunity tended to free me from man-made timetables and other societal strictures. I knew what it was to be alive because I knew it would not be forever. In this way I began to see one of the ultimate paradoxes of life—that it seems limitless when one realizes that the future in this form is limited.

Now, my journey has been long and filled with many experiences. My future in this body form grows shorter. The pace of time moves very quickly, and I want to make the most of it. When I was a child, the milestones I counted were the number of years that I had lived, and the future seemed boundless. Now that the limits draw near, I reckon time by how much is left.

Yes, time is all I have, and yet I do not have it either. I cannot possess this moment because it is mercurial and constantly in motion. It is as Einstein said: "For us believing physicists, this separation between past, present, and future has the value of mere illusion, however tenacious."

It is easy to become a time miser or a time squanderer, but I am warned by the words of Thoreau: "As if you could kill time without injuring eternity." I do not wish to be like the man Kierkegaard told of, who was so busy all of his life that he did not know he was alive until he died. I want to "use" my time wisely. That hour of play that my mother gave me as a child seemed endless. Now, the hours go before I know it. The months, years, decades go by. The young can afford to waste time; the old hold on to it. I want only to savor it—to move in its flow both carefully and trustingly.

2

Space

Good fences make good neighbors.

—Robert Frost

MY IRON LUNG was as much a part of me as my heart or liver, for I could not live without it. It was a vital organ. An electric power failure—and there were many at the military base where I first became ill—was more serious to me than a broken leg or a heart attack would have been. The iron lung was now my most personal and vital space boundary. It served as my new skin—this steel tank in which I was enclosed. In every sense it was personal, and nothing that happened to it or near it was without significance to me.

What I could see of myself revealed an unfamiliar configuration—not a human form, but a large steel cylinder painted yellow with chrome fittings. A noisy bellows rhythmically pumped life-giving air into me.

I could no longer make automatic responses. I could not have withdrawn my hand from a hot stove; I would only have a thought that I would like to. When I awakened from sleep, I could not spontaneously sit up. I was only aware of my desire to do so. My bladder and bowel functions were no longer automatic, in spite of the urges that I experienced. What was inside my body was as unfamiliar as what was outside. What I called myself before now seemed as foreign and enigmatic as a stranger in another country. What was me and mine was no longer clear, and my limits and boundaries seemed entirely arbitrary.

Intermittently people would open one or another of the portholes of my new metal skin and invade my private space. They would enter the most personal and private parts of me as they reached inside to move a leg or arm, or insert a needle or a bedpan. There was not even the pretense that my new space belonged to me, and entry beneath my new metal skin was at the discretion of others.

Those who attended to my body did things when and how they believed they should be done, and I seemed to have little or no part in this, except to feel the effect of what they did. They were not unkind, but they were more the owners of what lay inside the tank than I.

I was often cold. Lying still with no muscles that moved made it impossible for me to generate my own heat. So, shivering, I would call the nurse and ask for another blanket to cover me.

The room seemed comfortable to her, so she would doubt my judgment. In order to check, she would usually reach down to feel my leg. Then she would say something like "Oh, it's all right, you're not cold." Things like this happened over and over again. They thought they knew how *I* felt better than I did. I was not even acknowledged as a separate person. I would feel a blind rage rise within me. I felt as if the doctors, nurses, and orderlies were flaunting power over me by telling me I did not even know how I felt.

But you cannot get mad in hospitals. If you do, you may be in trouble. The next time you call for something, there may be a long delay in the nurses' response, or no response at all. There is always more than enough for the nurses to do in hospitals, so some things come first and some are left unattended. Angry patients come last.

So I quickly learned to smile patiently and attempt to explain that while I realized that a normal person would not find the room cool, I was shivering and uncomfortable. Even though no doubt she was correct in her objective judgment, if it would not be too much trouble, could she see if a blanket was available. I had to be very careful, for they were more in control of my body than I was.

There was one part of me that remained the same—my head. It protruded from one end of the iron lung and was the only part that remained recognizably human. People would address things to my head while they did other things to the iron lung and its contents. My head was treated as if it was separated from the rest of my body. People exchanged views with it as an equal, and they even asked permission before doing things to it.

Since my head continued to be familiar, and it was the only part that seemed to merit respect, I had fantasies, or perhaps they were hallucinations, of a surgical procedure that would separate the head so that it would be unencumbered by the body. Perhaps it could be reattached to another body, or simply kept alive by a machine. Such ideas now seem bizarre, but they seemed quite reasonable in the light of the confused understanding I had about what was me and what was not, which was my private space and which belonged to someone else.

Beyond the iron lung was my room. I was to spend a year there without leaving. This was the complete extent of the space about which I had firsthand knowledge. I heard reports from visitors and staff about what was happening outside my room—in the hospital, in the nearby towns, in the world, with my friends, with my family, and with others I knew. But all firsthand knowledge was about that ten-by-fifteen-foot room. Everything else was a matter of faith or fantasy—faith that what I was told was true or fantasy about what might be going on.

In spite of all this, I paradoxically continued to think of myself as the same person I had been. What I liked and disliked remained the same, and most of my thoughts had not changed greatly. The personal experiences that had formed my identity and history still lived in my mind. So it seemed to me that *I must* be the same person.

"Thought is born of failure," observed Lancelot Law Whyte. Indeed, when the smooth flow of action is blocked, thought is a means of finding resolution. When my physical activities were automatic, they required no conscious consideration. Now I had to look at myself and my life with new perspectives. My disability became my demanding teacher.

The wonder of how I existed in time was inextricably bound up with how I was in space. I had to cling to the most elemental definitions to maintain my sanity, because suddenly there were great changes inside my skin, and what had been so familiar now became alien. What I called myself, my "I," resided inside a body, a space-occupying mass that had been so familiar to me that it required no thought. Beyond my skin boundary was the outside world. Inside was me.

But my body, which I had called myself, had changed dramatically from autonomous to dependent, from strong to weak, from rapidly moving to completely immobile. I had to rely on others for even my most elemental functions and activities—even those that belonged in the bathroom. My spatial existence seemed more like that of a sack of flour than a human being.

Once, the six-year-old son of a friend put the whole matter in a nutshell. He had great difficulty categorizing me, for I seemed to have many of the privileges and responsibilities of an adult, but on the other hand, everything had to be done for me, as with a child. He did not know what to make of me. Finally, with a special joy that comes from insight and illumination, he said, "Oh, you're a big baby!" I did not share his joy over the category he placed me in, even though it did seem to fit.

I had been thrust backward in the developmental scale, and my dependence was now as profound as that of a newborn. Once again I had to deal with all of the overwhelming, degrading conditions of dependency that belong with infancy and childhood—at the same time that I considered myself a mature adult.

I did not adjust easily to my new dependence, and despised giving up what I had won years ago in long-forgotten battles. The baby and the man were in conflict, and the conflict was heightened by the many ways that other people treated me. Some people were interested in the dependent baby; others found the adult part, my head, more deserving of attention. Some seemed concerned with controlling what they considered the unruly child, while others wanted to nurture a helpless infant.

Nurses and attendants often talked to me as if I were a baby. If I became soiled through no fault of my own, they were likely to say, "Naughty, naughty," or "You've been a bad boy." Some people were so perplexed that they simply fled in despair. None of these attitudes helped clarify my confusion about how I thought of myself.

My body and the life I was actually living had changed, but my head, the repository of the past, had remained the same, so it caused me to wonder what really determined who I was. Was my identity determined by my head, by its relationship to my body, by the capacity or limitations of my body? Was it my past? None of these answers seemed entirely satisfying to me. Perhaps my identity depended on some mystical sense of myself in my mind.

There were also other aspects of my new relationship with space that I found disturbing. I spent nearly all of my time lying flat on my back, and from that position everyone seemed much taller and bigger. I could not judge the correct height of people, and sometimes my misjudgments were as much as a foot off. I once thought that a five-foot-four orderly was well over six feet tall. When I was not asking people what time it was, I was asking how tall they were.

Lying immobile on my back, I found that everything looked big and menacing. Even familiar things seemed strange. The taste of food that I had once enjoyed seemed different when it came at me from the hand of another, swooping down from above. I ate very little. Food did not seem right, even if it was something that in my mind, a moment before, seemed delicious.

Lying on your back is a wonderful position for rest or sleep, but it is not a good position from which to meet an unfamiliar and frightening world. All of my vulnerable parts were exposed, and I could do nothing to protect myself.

Since I could not move, one body position was as good as another. But it was not only the reality of positions that mattered, but the associations I had with various positions. Lying on my back was not a position I ever associated with being vigilant or able to defend myself. It is a perfectly terrible position in which to meet an attacker.

And that is how I perceived much of the contact that I had with people. I would often see their shadows before I saw them. They came at me from above like great condors, diving toward my exposed soft parts. People would capriciously and suddenly enter my most private spaces to do what was "best" for me. Since they did not ask my permission before doing things to me, they were like hostile invasions, and I felt violated. The savages had me cornered and were dancing threateningly about me with spears poised.

I had been on my back for a year, so the first time that I was placed in a wheelchair in a sitting position, I felt as though my power had been restored. I had far greater difficulty in breathing, and it lasted only three or four minutes. But who cared! It was position that counted, and I associated this one with being able to take care of myself.

My paralysis made gestures impossible, and I was amazed at how profoundly that compromised my ability to communicate subtlety. I could no longer convey mixed meanings or mute aggression by hand signals, and many jokes were completely impossible to tell without them. It is also hard to find a substitute for pointing to clarify direction, and it is hard to show resolve without standing firmly. As a result, I felt awkward when I spoke now, almost as though I were tongue-tied.

Directions presented special problems. Up and down ordinarily have a vertical frame of reference, but mine had changed from vertical to horizontal. To me, "move my arm up" meant toward my head and not toward the ceiling, as it was frequently interpreted. But more frustrating were right and left. Normal people often have trouble enough identifying their own sides, but on another person they are completely confused. My left leg was more often scratched when I had asked for my right, so I learned, for my own amusement, to patiently say, "That's good; now the other right one, please."

Although the hospital personnel frequently seemed to

invade me, people who visited seemed to keep an extra distance from me. They would leave more space than normal between us while we talked. When I would be introduced to someone new, they would hold back cautiously, so I rarely had physical contact with nonhospital people. They did not touch me, they did not shake my hand, they did not reach out in any physical way. They were probably afraid that they might hurt me, or catch what I had. Or perhaps they feared they might do something wrong and appear foolish. I was unable to reach out myself, so there remained a physical gulf between me and others in the world. It was lonely, and I longed to be touched. I sometimes thought that I was like a leper or an "untouchable."

Superstition can sometimes provoke an opposite reaction. Once I was out on the street, and a woman spotted me from the other side, made a right-angle turn, and walked directly over to me. Without a word she reached over and rubbed my back a couple of times, and then just as quickly started to leave. Confused, I asked, "Hey, what are you doing?" She just looked at me blankly and answered, "It's good luck if you touch a cripple." I asked, "For you or me?" She did not answer, and was gone.

It is strange that my first spatial concern was being invaded without my permission. Later, I was dismayed that people seemed to stay away from me entirely. Just as other people felt awkward with me, so did I with them. Either way, my boundaries were insecure and I felt off balance. Fear of rejection or of appearing foolish by intruding where I was not wanted kept me from initiating physical contact by use of words. Slowly, however, I began to realize that the responsibility was mine, and I had to do things to make physical contact easier.

When I began to try to overcome this physical gulf, I found my efforts were rejected very rarely. Usually people were relieved and grateful when I let them know what I wanted them to do. As I have become more open and less embarrassed about myself, the chasms seem to have lessened. My fears that others might not respond, or worse, would respond unwillingly, are seldom realized.

We avoid and fear the unknown. Indeed, it may be filled with horrible dangers, but maybe, just maybe you can soar into the heavens. Perhaps that is what we fear—becoming untethered in flight—and so we prefer instead to be grounded to the past miseries; they are at least secure and fastened down.

A human being is loath to give up what he has learned, even if it no longer fits the present reality. He resists acquiring the new, even when its advantages are clear. The old and accustomed may be moribund, but the new must have time to be born.

I have met a lot of people who were unwilling to give up the past and who treasured it as a miser covets gold. If the past is filled with pleasure—"my mother loved me"; "I was the best cheerleader at school"; "you should have seen me the time I ran for that touchdown"—it's easy to understand. Less understandable is someone who clings to events that are only painful—"I can't get her out of my mind, she was so awful"; "I hate him as much today as I did then"; and "I keep thinking of it over and over again, it was the worst experience of my life." When the only choices are between the obsolete past and the unknown future, many people prefer to hold onto the past, even though it was miserable.

I was taught in medical school that the brain was the organ of the mind and that the body represented reality. However powerful the mind is, it is an expression of the body. This may be only half true. Perhaps it is the other way around too and how I exist in space is also an expression of my mind. Certainly my beliefs seem to play a stronger role in how I experience life than reality does. Is the only possible disability a disability of the mind, then? Is my reluctance to take on new beliefs and attitudes, to assume the impossible, also my resistance to the freedom of soaring beyond what I know?

Even though I am severely physically disabled, the feeling of well-being that I sometimes have now is just as intense as it was when I was called healthy. In those moments of well-being, it is entirely a matter of my focus of attention. I seem to have no illness when I am unaware of what limits me and can see only the horizons that I aim for.

Of course, what I was taught in medical school may still be true, and my lack of awareness of my body does not mean that it is not still telling my mind what to do. But who am I really? Am I a body that has a brain, which in turn has a mind? Or am I a mind that uses a body for certain purposes? There seems to be something of me, some part of me that is not grounded, not attached to my body, for it moves through time at a different pace.

When I lose my sense of myself and am fully involved with something I value or someone I love, my body seems to become irrelevant, and my boundaries seem to include the other thing or person. There seems no distinction between us. It is as though, at those moments, my boundaries include everything—the whole universe.

When I am aware of my body, it is because some special experience has drawn my attention to it. I experience pain or pleasure from inside it. I experience movement or contact when I bump into another person or something. However, when I join with some other person or task and am fully absorbed, it is as though I have left my body and am but a pinpoint of awareness—aware only of this moment and this "thing."

There is a magical quality to these moments. Time and space are fused, and my body seems to disappear. Time accelerates, so that I am identified with it, and I am time. At these moments, my space seems to be the universe.

The ambiguities of what is real in space and time give me hope, or perhaps faith, that there is something larger and more important than what I am in this limited space. While I cannot fully grasp what that is, I find comfort in assuming that there is reason to recognize this something larger.

When I am able to bring my space-time relationships into synchrony, when my mind and my body seem to move at the same pace, I feel whole and alive again. When the discrepancy is wide, it is like terror or death. Who I am in this moment between life and death is what I believe I am, and what I believe I am allows some room for choice.

3

Relationships

A human being is part of the whole, called by us "universe," a part limited in time and space. He experiences himself, his thoughts and feelings as something separate from the rest—a kind of optical delusion of his consciousness. This delusion is a kind of prison for us, restricting us to our personal decisions and to affection for a few persons nearest to us. Our task must be to free ourselves from this prison by widening our circle of compassion to embrace all living creatures and the whole of nature in its beauty.

—Albert Einstein

A S WE KNOW, time and space are relative concepts in physics; solid matter can be turned into energy, and energy is transformed to matter under certain conditions. The state of any one thing depends on its relationships to others. My awareness of time-space relativity was confirmed by new personal experience, and especially by my relationships with other people.

At times I felt as if I had lost my human qualities, and did not belong to the species *Homo sapiens* any longer. I felt like one of the sacks of produce I used to carry at one of my jobs. When I looked at my motionless hands, I saw a bunch of bananas. I had become a "thing."

As an inanimate object, I was in constant need of attention and care from human beings. My most private and personal functions rested in the hands of others. I was a Martian dependent on Earthlings for my survival.

I had no words that could adequately describe what I felt. I was exposed utterly and completely. I was vulnerable to everyone and everything. Nothing was private; there was only wordless shame for what I had become. Logic and rationality were useless to me.

These overwhelming feelings greatly sensitized me to those who cared for me. I scrutinized the countenance of my attendants for their every mood and whim. Everything that affected them affected me. If I was cared for willingly and without reluctance, I felt good and the world was sunny. If my care was given grudgingly or irritably, in a callous way, powerful feelings of degradation swept over me.

This helped me to understand something I read much later about the effectiveness of the brainwashing techniques used by North Koreans and Chinese during the Korean war.

Many people were puzzled and perplexed at the astonishing number of captured Americans who embraced the ideology of their captors. But I could understand when I learned the nature of some of the most effective and diabolical of the brainwashing techniques. All personal care and functioning was carefully controlled and used to reward and punish. The opportunity for urination and defecation was at the caprice of the captors. When they were allowed bathroom privileges, the captives' hands and feet were bound, so that any preparation necessary for urination or defecation was literally in the hands of the captors. The prisoners' feeling of dependence was so urgent that they became sensitized to every mood and whim of the guards. As a result, many of the soldiers accepted their guards' ideology, although it was completely alien to what they had believed before.

The captive Americans had a way out. They could embrace the ideology of their captors. But my dilemma was different, for nothing that I could do would restore me to grace. Although I depended entirely on how my "captors" felt and behaved for my self-esteem, I could never become one of them—no matter how hard I tried to please them.

Some of the people I depended on made it clear that it was "just a job" to them.

In one hospital, the first hour of the nurses' shift was spent in a detailed discussion of who would take coffee breaks when. Medications, patient needs, all other things paled in comparison. Sometimes people would literally leave you in midair in a lift to go on a coffee break, or leave you in some other awkward position, and just say, "It's my break time." They would often do everything possible to avoid helping me. What they did was done in a perfunctory manner. They seemed reluctant or grudging as they did things. There was a guardedness about them, fearing that they would be asked to do more than they were willing or able to do.

One of the worst times was at "change of shift," what seemed like an interminable period when all nursing staff from two shifts would gather together to review doctors' orders and "progress notes." During that time there was absolutely no chance of getting anyone to help you, no matter how urgent the problem.

I was on a ward with thirty patients, most of whom were as helpless as I. Watching all those nurses through the glass of the nursing station was like looking through the window of a candy store. We could see what we urgently wanted, but there was no way of getting it. We would wait expectantly to see who would ultimately be assigned to our ward.

If it was "Ivan the Terrible," we knew we were in trouble. Ivan, as we called him, was always attired in heavy black boots. He would stand at one end of the hallway with his hands on his hips, legs apart, menacingly surveying his charges. No one dared speak or ask for anything. Then he would walk to the center of the room to make his daily pronouncement: "I worked too hard yesterday, and I ain't doin' nothing today." Whereupon he would stride dramatically out of the room.

He would not return until ward rounds began a couple of hours later, when the doctors and nurses would go through the wards together. Then, psychopath that he was, Ivan would appear, all smiles, to join them in making rounds.

Fearful of reprisal, we patients would diplomatically try to explain our most urgent unattended needs. If the doctors and nurses were the least bit surprised or irritated that Ivan had not done his job and ordered him to give this patient a bedpan or that one a bath, he would be in an angry mood, and then you were in for some rough handling.

Others were nicknamed "Leona the Late" because she always was, and "Ed the Reluctant," so named because whatever request was made of him, he had to go someplace else first and usually would not return at all. They may have been the worst of our "keepers," but on a normal distribution curve they would not be too far off center.

To me, what they did or did not do was not "just a job," but a matter of survival, of both my physical body and my sense of myself as a person. With callous helpers I felt especially like an undeserving outsider—regarded at best with curiosity, but usually with disinterest or disdain. Yet pity was no better. Feelings of humiliation would sweep over me at such times.

Fortunately there was another sort of helper. Just thinking about them now I become warm and relaxed. These people helped willingly, with interest and compassion. They seemed to receive something valuable from the act of giving. My comfort was their goal. When one of them would appear on a ward of patients, it was as though the room would suddenly light up. Fear and tension would recede.

These willing helpers were among the most appealing people I have ever met. They seemed happy, generous, open, and compassionate. They were nurtured by their relationships with people who needed them. They usually had a remarkable sensitivity to the needs of people as well, often seeming to understand without words.

With them I felt restored to the human community. They seemed to welcome me back as they supported the best in me. Their generosity transformed both those they helped and themselves into richer, fuller human beings.

M.J., a physical therapist, was an example. She was always willing to help with whatever you needed, whether it fell within her "job description" or not. It was enough that you were in need and she could help. It was over thirty years ago when I first met her on a hospital ward, and she is still my friend. You do not forget people like her.

Glen Holmes was a doctor who, observing that I needed a shave, voluntarily gave me one when he had the time. When the power went out, he was the first one there to manually pump my iron lung.

I was fascinated to learn that many of these helpful people had grown up in families with a severely disabled member for whom they had been partly responsible. Some had disabled parents, others disabled siblings. There were others who had to work as children in concert with others in the family, on small farms or in a family business. They seemed to realize that their lives were inextricably bound with the lives of others.

These compassionate helpers who seemed to ask for nothing got a great deal. I was always eager to see them, and their generosity made me feel generous, in both practical matters and emotional expression. I felt as though I had something to give them. When they were in bad moods, I would reach out to them. They would share their trials and sadness at times, and get support from me.

The responsiveness of these compassionate helpers made me feel human again, and brought forth the qualities in me that made it possible to be a support to others. With them I felt returned from exile. The pariah was forgiven for his crime, and felt restored to life.

Those who give grudgingly are the unlucky ones. Their guardedness divides them from other people, so they get little back. They must feel like outsiders with most people. Their guardedness also divides them from themselves, producing tension, and tension is the enemy of health and well-being. They feel they have so little to give that they must be stingy.

Of course, most people who helped me were at neither extreme, and even the most compassionate had bad days, and occasionally the worst of the attendants had good ones. They had the variety of moods and feelings of all human beings.

It is hard to give, much less give generously, if you feel that you do not have enough. But stinginess produces deficiency; withholding causes others to withhold, and in the end the person who thinks he does not have enough to give is deprived.

I learned something more about stinginess and generosity too. Getting enough air, being able to go to the bathroom when necessary, having enough food and rest are urgent needs, and I could do none of these elemental things for myself. When those needs were not met, I could not be compassionate to someone else. There is no opportunity for higher levels of human function when you are short of air, and all that you can think of is getting the next breath. I am not good for anything else unless these needs are met.

But here is the remarkable thing. The urgency with which I experience my needs depends on the confidence I have that they *can* be met, whether they are or not. They are not so urgent when I am surrounded by people who willingly help me if called upon. But if I am in unfamiliar circumstances, or with people whom I know cannot be depended upon, I can think of little else but those primitive physiological needs.

When I feel confident that those around me *would* be willing to help if asked, I feel rather relaxed about it. I am willing to subordinate my needs to something which they need. I am willing to wait my turn because I know it will come, and while waiting, I am able and willing to reach out with some compassion.

So most of the time even what I have thought of as physiological needs are relative, and depend on the friendliness and nourishment of the surroundings. My attitudes and level of consciousness are transformed to higher levels and more affirmative thoughts when I am surrounded by those who have the same thoughts and attitudes. If those around me view the world guardedly, as a place of deficiencies, I adopt that attitude as well.

In fact, most of the people who surround us are not so different from us.

Although my mother and father lived hard lives, I think they did as well as any. They had escaped the persecutions of Eastern Europe and come to a new and sometimes forbidding land where they had to struggle against harsh conditions, strange language and customs, sometimes exploitations and prejudice. But they were not embittered, and always maintained gratitude for what they had and the hope that things could get better. No one is adequately prepared for hardship, but the groundwork they laid was as good as any.

My disability has shown me that I am not so separate from others, and I have come to see with increasing clarity that there is synchrony on all levels between people. We are neither as independent nor as autonomous as we have believed. The independence that I once prized I now realize was in part a luxury that I could indulge myself in because of self-deception. My eyes can deceive me into believing that I am separate from others, but when I admit awareness derived from other people's senses, I realize how closely we are related.

My kinship is not limited to those with my bloodlines, but is open to all those with whom I have contact. The more open my attitude is, and the more I am able to lower my guard, the more I create a spirit of kinship, as well as receive it.

My immediate personal experience confirms that physical and mental health and well-being, stress reduction and elevation of consciousness, all of the things that I strive for, are enhanced by openness and generosity toward others, and theirs toward me.

Einstein transformed our knowledge of the physical properties of objects: that they do not stand alone and their form depends on relationships in time and space. Humans are even more dependent on their relationships with one another. But most of us suffer from what he calls an "optical delusion," in which we believe we are separate. This keeps us from the "compassion to embrace all living creatures and the whole of nature in its beauty."

"Kindness" has the same etymology as "kinship." In

their ancient meanings they formed one concept, implying that you behave in a kind manner toward those "of the same kind." When a person behaves kindly, he enlarges the scope of his kinship relationships and promotes the strengths of all of us.

Not long before his death, Aldous Huxley made this observation: "It's a bit embarrassing to have been concerned with the human problem all one's life and to find at the end that one has no more to offer by way of advice than 'try to be a little kinder.'"

I can understand Huxley's embarrassment and Einstein's modesty, for what my disability has shown me, and what their unique, scholarly perspectives had shown them, is but the ancient wisdom: that you get what you give. Goodwill begets goodwill, and openness produces openness.

There is something in the nature of our perception and in our capacity for rational thought which produces the optical delusion of which Einstein spoke. It is only from the most revered sources and, if we are lucky, from our own experience that we find the larger view.

Our view of dependency is generally that it is a weakness and a flaw. There is a special pride one derives from feeling independent. It is a position that we have valued and taught. But I have come to a different understanding of the meaning of dependence and independence.

Every living being depends on others of its kind and the environment for nourishment and support. So a feeling of independence is not based on a belief that one is self-sufficient, but on a confidence that what one needs *is* available from the outside. The wider the circle that we can rely upon, the more we can feel and behave independently.

We confuse this feeling of independence with self-sufficiency, and interpret it to mean that we have done everything on our own. The belief that we are "self-made" men and women is a belief in a biological impossibility. That is the optical delusion of which Einstein spoke.

The more a person believes he must rely on himself alone or on just a few others, the more he behaves penuriously. He has all of his eggs in one basket, and so must cling tightly to what he has. His independence is under constant siege, and his brittle self-esteem is continuously on the line if the circle of his dependence is small.

Disability has forced me to see beyond the optics of the situation and to see how closely related I am to others. I am dependent on the supplies and moods of other people, of nature, of all things. Their fate becomes my fate. I must find ways of nurturing them, so they can nurture me.

We live amidst a cosmic irony. I am forced to experience myself as the center of this universe. I can see the world only from my perspective. Everyone else is imprisoned in the same way, perceiving the world from his or her perspective. In this limitless system any point can be perceived as the center. But still, the evidence is unmistakable. We are all connected, and parts of one whole. We are not alone, even if our eyes tell us we are.

My quest must be to find a way of entering that consciousness which will allow me to see both my perspective and the larger one at the same time. The few glimpses that I have had of that elevated plane show me its truth. But when I look back at those moments to see how I got there, the trail has disappeared, and I have to start afresh.

4

Reconstruction

There is no surprise more magical than the surprise of being loved. It is God's finger on man's shoulder.

—Charles Morgan, *The Fountain*

I GOT SICK on a Friday the thirteenth. I had never been superstitious before, but that certainly caused me to wonder. Yogi Berra once said about superstitions, "I don't know, but why take a chance?" I share Berra's ambivalence. So since then, whenever I see a Friday the thirteenth coming up on the calendar, I cautiously avoid taking any chances.

I did seem star-crossed. First, the Navy recalled me from the reserve to active duty. When I reported, they pronounced me physically fit and gave me new orders. Bizarre as it seems, my new orders were to go on duty with the Army. During the Korean War the Navy had plenty of doctors, while the Army did not have enough. So I was given a new set of orders to go to an Army station in Texas. But en route I got sick, and went to the nearest military hospital.

Then, nobody wanted me. The Navy said I was not their responsibility; the Army said I was not theirs. The Veterans Administration said that my illness was not service-connected, and I did not belong to them either.

Hence, I was not eligible for any benefits. They even stuck me with the cost of the new uniforms and they did not reimburse me for my travel.

As irrational as it seemed to me, it was all clear to the military mind. In its wisdom the Navy had concluded that the incubation period for polio was twenty-one days, despite the research that clearly showed that it can vary from a few hours to as long as six months. So although I was under orders when I reported, bought uniforms, and traveled, and although I was physically examined and pronounced fit, they now said I was not in the Navy at all. If that was so, where *had* I been? The Navy made me disappear by an act of magic, one that would have been a credit to Houdini. Ironically, if I had not obeyed those orders, I would have been arrested. "There's a right way, a wrong way, and a Navy way, and we do it in the Navy way."

The Navy specializes in creating that sort of irrationality. Another example occurred shortly after I entered the naval hospital as a patient (which, of course, according to the Navy, hadn't happened). The temperature outside was close to 100 degrees. Inside, the furnaces suddenly and inexplicably went on. To everyone's consternation the heat remained on all day, producing several cases of heat stroke. The puzzle was solved the next day. We learned that the commandant of naval hospitals was stationed in Alaska. It was cold there in the fall, and since one directive from him covered all hospitals, the heat went on in San Diego too. In semitropical Southern California the hottest weather of the year usually occurs in the fall, but there were no excep-

48 · *Flying Without Wings*

tions in the Navy, and when the commandant ordered heat, we all got heat.

When I first entered a naval hospital I was not yet paralyzed, so the diagnosis of "nonparalytic polio" was made. Within a few hours I had become completely paralyzed, but they never changed the diagnosis. I did think, wryly—as I lay in an iron lung unable to move at all—that if what I had was the nonparalytic form, I was sure glad I did not get the more serious paralytic one.

So it was in the eyes of the Navy: I had not gone on duty, and therefore had not been recalled, and according to my records (which did not exist) my polio had been nonparalytic, so it was only reasonable that the Navy now recall me to the active duty to which I had actually reported.

At regular intervals I would receive new orders from the Navy Department telling me to report immediately to this or that facility for active duty. At first I would responsibly have someone telegraph back, describing my situation. My responses were never acknowledged, but then in a few months entirely new orders would come to me. After a time I began to realize the uselessness of responding to the orders, and anyway, there really was not much they could do to me if I just ignored them, so I stopped answering.

The Navy does not give up easily, however, and the orders continued to come for years. Finally I began to receive threats that if I did not report, grave consequences would occur. Then at last they spelled out the grave consequences: if I did not report, they would discharge me from the service. Finally they did send me a discharge certificate, thus completing the illusion.

The amazing thing to me is that we won World War II.

I am indebted to the Navy for the laughs I got after I became accustomed to this incredible behavior. But there was also a very serious problem. I had no money, and my last job had been as an intern, where my salary had been ten dollars per month plus board and room. (In those days, the better the internship, the less it paid.)

Then came the good luck. The March of Dimes came to my rescue. The national foundation was begun by President Franklin Roosevelt, himself a polio victim, to care for others with the disease. Very few people were in a position to pay for the lengthy hospital rehabilitation required. The foundation generously paid for all of my care, after the Army, Navy, and VA gave up on me, and it was excellent care.

Now that polio has been nearly completely eradicated, it is easy to forget what a fearful specter it was to children, the usual victims, and their parents. The near-panic led to tremendous public support that enabled the foundation to pay for the care of every victim who needed it.

Just how lucky I was became apparent when I met patients at the hospital who had diseases that were not subsidized. For example, Guillain-Barré syndrome can have the same paralyzing effects as polio. So there were people in the hospital who had symptoms almost identical to mine but could not share the benefits of the March of Dimes, even though they needed care as much as I did. I had already learned that life was not fair, but this time I was one of the fortunate ones.

Gradually, with time and therapy, I became stronger. Although I still could not walk or stand, I was able to breathe longer on my own. I could also sit upright in my wheelchair for nearly an hour at a time, and if things were placed in just the right positions, I could move my hand enough to write my name.

I could see that I could not expect much more improvement, and I began to think seriously about what I was going to do with my life. Fortunately I had finished my basic medical training. But what could I do with it? Could I find a specialty the physical demands of which did not exceed my abilities? The most sedentary specialties were dermatology, pathology, and radiology, but all of them required physical activity that was beyond my capacity. Of all specialties, psychiatry had the fewest physical demands and seemed the most logical. The major vehicle is talking, and my speech was one thing that, with the exception of volume, was relatively unimpaired. There was little of a physical nature that was required of a psychiatrist, particularly in those days. I also had considerable interest in the field, although I had been turned off by some poor teaching early in my career.

My decision was aided also by a bit of good luck. An extraordinary young woman was one of the few patients at the hospital, like me, who continued to require an iron lung. We did not see or speak to one another because of our immobility, but we heard about each other. Her husband and legions of friends and family visited regularly. When she was busy with her care, her guests would visit sometimes with me. Her husband was also a tennis player and a successful business executive. We became friends, and I developed great respect for him. When he encouraged me to enter psychiatry, I took it very seriously. I also met several psychiatrists among their circle of friends, and got further encouragement.

They also helped to reintroduce me to the world, a forbidding place when you've been hospitalized and away from it for nearly three years. My first live meeting with the woman I had come to know so much about from others occurred when she and her husband took me to dinner at a restaurant. To be out in public was a major step for someone like me who had been isolated in a hospital for years, and they made it easy.

When we entered, it seemed as though all eyes were on me, as if daring the pariah to invade the domain of those who belonged. But my protectors reassured me and behaved as though I had every right to be there.

I will always be grateful to that couple for their thoughtfulness. They even bought me my first wheelchair, a new model not yet offered by the March of Dimes.

Standard wheelchairs either did not recline or did so only partially. In order to breathe I had to lie nearly flat most of the time, making my new wheelchair a necessity. It would allow me to be easily moved from lying down to upright and back again.

So once again I was forced to consider the nature of kinship. The kind people to whom you feel closest are not necessarily kin in the sense of the same family. But you can feel related for many different reasons.

Living on a ward with thirty severely disabled male polio patients presents powerful realities. One is the need for stretching. A major problem with polio rehabilitation is that damaged or destroyed muscles are replaced by fibrous tissues, causing shortening and contractures. Those muscles must be regularly stretched, an extremely painful procedure which can be likened to the medieval torture known as "the rack." A physical therapist manually forces a shortened muscle group to reach what would be normal range of motion.

Another reality is what is on the minds of young confined men: food and sex. Food is mentioned to complain how bad it is: "They ought to fire the dietician and hire a cook." Of course, missed most of all by a deprived group of men are women and sex. Despite the paralysis, in polio the senses and sexual functions are not impaired. So any unsuspecting young woman who entered the ward was likely to be the subject of elaborate fantasy and discussion. As the man in the next bed often remarked, "I'm ready, willing, and *unable*."

Stretching and sex were dramatically brought together on those days when the physical therapy department assigned Rita to do the stretching on the ward. Among the young physical therapists, occupational therapists, and nurses in the hospital, many were very attractive young women, but Rita stood out among them all. Slender and graceful, she perfectly filled out her starched white uniform. Raven tresses fell to her shoulders, and her deep brown eyes emphasized her patrician features.

Among her most appealing qualities was how she unassumingly ignored the whistles and innuendos which understandably came her way. She took her responsibilities very seriously and simply and purposefully went about her business. She gave no quarter when she stretched, taking a stretch to the limit of the patient's tolerance, knowing just the right point at which to stop.

A joke on the ward was that "the definition of mixed emotions is being stretched by Rita," implying that the pleasure of seeing her was mixed with the pain of stretching. Another wag described the experience as the "essence of masochism." All of the joking was in good humor, and not a man on the ward would have traded his time with Rita for any other activity during the day.

At the time I was both surprised by and mistrustful of any evidence of interest in me by young women. I thought it proved that there was something wrong with them, as implied in Groucho Marx's famous saying: "I wouldn't want to belong to any club that would have me as a member." I had so many self-doubts, and was so embarrassed about my body, that I was very afraid of disclosing myself. So I kept my relationships with women rather superficial and impersonal.

Although I was very attracted to Rita, I did not dare to let her know, even when she, ordinarily very businesslike and somewhat shy, showed evidence of friendliness toward me. At first I mistrusted my own perceptions. But then I could not ignore that something more might be happening when she would, from time to time, drop by on her way home to say good night.

We were like two wary scouts, saying very little, restraining all expression of affection to one another, while at the same time attempting to read all possible significance into the utterings of the other. I doubted what I noticed, and she suppressed what she felt.

About this time I had a serious setback, one of the frequent accompaniments of polio. Inactivity can lead to the demineralization of bones, and this can produce kidney stones. I developed one, and had to be transferred to an acute hospital for a couple of weeks.

On my way out on the gurney, in severe pain, feeling even worse about myself than usual and wishing no one would see me, Rita suddenly appeared, kissed me reassuringly on the cheek, and patted my shoulder. During those two agonizing weeks I was in the acute hospital, I was sustained by the memory of what she had done. I went over and over it in my mind. Could it be the lovely Rita was interested in me? (She later confided in me that she was engaged in a struggle similar to mine, with thoughts such as "Oh God, don't let me fall in love with him.")

The doubts that I had were dispelled when I returned, for now she openly told me that she missed me and thought of me. A few weeks later she told me that she and her roommate, one of the nursing staff, had rented an apartment nearby, and I was invited to be a guest—her guest—on a weekend when her roommate would be away.

Rita was Boston, Italian, Catholic; I was California, beach and tennis, Jewish. Yet we seemed to have a special bond. There was something alike about us—so much so that several times we were mistaken for brother and sister.

We spent a lot of time talking and just "hanging out." We played backgammon and bridge. We liked to move around and travel to see things. At first, before we had a car, we would walk; that is, Rita would push me. And we did a lot of exploring, sometimes doing things you wouldn't believe. I've been in the surf in my wheelchair with Rita (ruining the wheelchair). We both come from families where food was important. Rita is a gourmet chef, and I am interested in recipes as well, and we used to experiment a lot, particularly for guests. There is a certain mutuality which brought us together. I told stories and jokes, and I loved to hear her laugh. She, I think, used to particularly enjoy doing things for me, as she could see the response of making me happy. The mutual positive influence was especially rewarding.

But in spite of the things that seemed to bring us together, one big thing separated us. I was in love with someone else.

That someone else was me, or rather my image of what I used to be. My past was my standard, and I carried it with me like a Pepsi generation commercial. And, of course, I assumed that everyone else, including Rita, was attracted to that same image. So naturally Rita, in my mind, had to find the legions of other young men who were interested in her more appealing. My closed system excluded any alternative views.

What Rita saw in me was not what I saw, however. All of my physical problems, which seemed in the forefront to me, were background issues for her, "minor inconveniences," as she said. She was not oblivious to their significance; she just did not see them as important as other things. For me, her views created puzzlement, sometimes irritation, sometimes dismay, and sometimes, even occasionally, love.

She was ruled by the heart, enjoyed being with me, and so it "felt right" to her. That was enough for her. Her head told her she should date others, and she did, then ended up wishing she had stayed around the hospital with me. She was as optimistic about our relationship as I was pessimistic. We talked of marriage, but it always came down to the same thing for me. I did not know how long I was going to live. I did not know if I would ever work again, and to take on new responsibilities in which I might fail would only make me feel worse.

At the same time I continued to move toward work and career plans. I applied to countless programs for residency training in psychiatry. Most programs did not even answer after learning of my physical condition. Some straightforwardly rejected me, and a few left the door open. The program directors were physicians, but they are not, I discovered, immune to awkwardness in dealing with a disabled person. I got one interview with a program director who evidently had not read the description of my physical limitations on my application, or it just did not register. When I entered his office he just stared at me, seemingly thunderstruck. I introduced myself and told him of my interest in training; he continued to look at me as though I had just flown in on a flying saucer. Then he arose from his chair and abruptly said, "I have an appointment," and left the room without further explanation. I waited there a while, and then concluded that our interview must be over and he was not coming back until I left. So I did, feeling crushed and isolated. He simply did not know what to do with me.

The chairman of the Psychiatry Department at my school, Stanford, was about as bad. He responded with effusive friendliness, but complete obfuscation, until I had to give up. I felt more comfortable with interviewers who were candid. If they pressed me for details of how I would handle the physical and psychological demands, their candor enlarged my awareness of the problems. I did get accepted by one of the best residency programs in the country. However, they were not sure that I could make it, and offered me a position without pay. But I needed money desperately since I had nothing to live on.

Then I lucked out. A new program was starting at a state hospital, and they had not yet selected residents. I got an appointment to meet with the hospital director, who sat impassively listening, while his two associates tried to persuade me it was hopeless for me to work there. I tried to convince them I could do it. Then the director spoke for the first time. "I don't think we ought to discourage this young man," he said. Suddenly all sorts of possibilities opened up. I realized that he was the source of all power in that institution. He knew every detail, and ruled with a benevolent hand. The staff had to follow his expectations, and could act only at his behest. I later learned that all letters that were sent from that hospital were personally read and approved by him. He was very demanding, but I will always be grateful to old Dr. Wyers for giving me a chance.

So one day at the hospital where I was a patient, they got me up, shaved me, took me to the bathroom, dressed me, put me in my reclining wheelchair, lifted me into my brother's car, and folded up my wheelchair, and my brother drove me forty miles to the state hospital, where I started work. I saw my first patient an hour after I arrived.

Residency training in psychiatry requires three years of specialized clinical education and experience in hospital, clinic, and community settings. You work as a psychiatrist under supervision while attending seminars and courses. After three years, you must work for two more in a supervised setting. Then, after those five years, you are eligible to be examined for certification by the American Board of Psychiatry and Neurology.

While in training you are a doctor, and have to do all the physical things doctors do. Despite my limitations, with the help of an attendant I could do a creditable physical examination on my patients, with a few exceptions. I had to rely on my colleagues to do pelvic and rectal exams for me.

My salary was $295 per month. I had advertised in the newspaper for an attendant with a car who would take care of me twenty-four hours a day, seven days a week, for $200 per month, plus board and room. We would live temporarily at my brother's house, which was close to the hospital.

I had three attendants in the first three weeks. All day and then all night was just too much for them. I was in a panic, not knowing where or how they might leave. The selections I made were inappropriate, and my expectations were unrealistic. In addition, I was becoming increasingly uncomfortable, because I could see that I was disrupting my brother's household.

That was a very bad period for me: not certain who would take care of me, guilty about where I was living, starting a new profession with rusty skills and many new ones I had to acquire, while trying to find innovative ways of dealing with my disability. Nothing seemed secure or reliable.

The only respite came on the weekends, when Rita would come to visit. Everything suddenly turned easy then. When she cared for me, it seemed effortless and a part of some other, more interesting activity. What I paid my two-hundred-pound male attendants to do while grunting and groaning with agony, she did as naturally and as unobtrusively as though I were not even disabled.

As she had predicted, my big problems were minor inconveniences when she was there. So, against the odds, we got married by a judge one weekend, me in my reclining wheelchair, alternately lying flat and sitting up, feeling like the creature from outer space, and Rita in her usual radiant naturalness.

Our combined assets, with wedding presents, were somewhat less than $1,000. We rented a furnished house for $100 per month in a small Chicano ghetto not too far from the hospital. I continued to have an attendant drive me to work in his car and help me during the day. I paid him $200 per month, without board and room.

Rita got a job working part-time as a clerk in a nearby city hall. Since we had no car, she had to take the bus. She initially made just over $1.00 per hour, about average in 1953. When Rita was not working, she was taking care of me and our little house. In those days I was not yet appropriately in awe of what she was able to do. I was too preoccupied with my fatigue and the demands on me to notice. How she did it, I do not know.

Despite all that I have described, it was a very happy time for us. We both worked hard, up to our capacities. We had good neighbors and friends, and we laughed a lot. Laughter was wonderful. Even today, no pleasure is so great for me as when Rita breaks into laughter, particularly if I had had some part in causing it to happen.

After six months it appeared to the hospital director that I was going to survive, and that I might even turn out to be a pretty good resident. So they doubled my salary and offered us a small house on the hospital grounds for less than half of what we were paying nearby. Quite a bonanza!

This was an old-style state hospital, where patients stayed a long time and were given work assignments at the hospital farm, in the dairy, in the power station, with the fire department, and so on. Helping me became one such assignment, one of the most popular in the hospital among the patients, and it added to the stability of my life.

Rita had a little breathing room for the first time. I was away at work for at least eight hours a day, often more, and she no longer had to go to work herself. She could be a real housewife full-time. In a couple of months we bought our first car, a sporty 1953 Delray Chevrolet. It looked like my survival was promising, we were going to make it as a married couple, and there even seemed to be a future ahead of us.

In times of war you deal only with survival issues. When the war ends, you find there are still problems you had not been paying attention to. They may have been insignificant before; now they become more urgent. My physical problems were wartime survival issues. However, now we had the luxury to worry about those second-tier problems.

Some minor inconveniences to me were big issues to Rita. She had very strong feelings about the aesthetics of all things—home arrangements, decorations, food, and clothing (including mine)—things that were for me fairly unimportant. Rita usually could not find her keys—a minor detail for her, a big deal for me. If I got angry, she got mad at me for getting mad. All of our differences could now be allowed to surface.

We then discovered that talking and silence had different meanings for us. My family engaged in a great deal of talking and discussion about everything as I grew up. The only time there was silence was when somebody was angry at somebody else. Those were chilly, uncomfortable moments. In Rita's family, by contrast, the best moments were in silence, when there was no criticism being exchanged. So I misinterpreted her silence as anger, and she found my need to discuss things irritating. The great thing was that we were now just like any other married couple, learning to live with differences.

Having hospital patients as attendants to help me was a mutually rewarding experience, although at times strange and occasionally frightening. It gave the patients something useful to do; expectations were not too high, there was a certain status attached to working with a doctor, and of course they earned some money.

One of the great advantages of this arrangement was the overlapping of roles between doctor and patient, helper and person in need. I helped them, they helped me, and we were friends. This balanced my training, which emphasized the importance of the doctor/patient role differences and the use of structure and role in practice. Indeed, I have a healthy respect for the importance of structure, but I will always be grateful that my relationships with patient/helpers kept me from slipping into rigid role relationships that can so easily dehumanize people. People who are hungry to relate may be put off by an inaccessible doctor, and feel unworthy of more equal relationships.

My helpers often helped me to see reality with clearer eyes. Arthur, one of my early helpers, was a strange, chaotic young man who had attempted to strangle his girlfriend when he interpreted her actions as evidence that she thought him homosexual. Our conversations were mainly about food, but contained powerful metaphorical overtones. He would tell me what he ate at each meal. For example, he had reported having tuna casserole. I asked how it was. He responded, thoughtfully, with something like "Well, it was pretty good once you stopped looking for the tuna." He was always gravely humorless, but full of philosophical wisdom. Arthur was just reporting reality as he saw it, and he saw it naked, without its customary cover. He was correct—you would not be disappointed if you were not wedded to your expectations. It was, of course, the very lesson he and I needed to learn.

Then there was Joe, a catatonic schizophrenic who rarely spoke and who would just look blankly at you. He willingly did what I asked of him, and although he hardly spoke at all, we had a relationship of sorts. Occasionally he surprised me. Once, when we entered the ward with the most disturbed patients, a wild-looking man rushed at me, angrily demanding that I get out of my wheelchair and stand up. I tried to explain that I could not, but this made him angrier. He seized my arm and began pulling me out of the chair, uttering something insane about devil possession, killing the son of God, and he was Jesus—all in an unintelligible jumble.

I was really scared, and it looked as though I could not count on Joe, who seemed involved in his own hallucinations. Suddenly Joe's voice boomed out, loud and adamant, "Don't be stupid; he's crippled!" My wild assailant was startled, and stopped. He looked at Joe, then at me, and. said, "Oh, I'm sorry," and then began helping me get back in my wheelchair.

I started to thank Joe, but realized that the effort of speaking had taken too much out of him and that he had already retreated to his inner world. He eventually did get better, well enough to leave the hospital, and the last I heard he was living with his sister, though not yet employed regularly.

There were many such experiences, filled with fear, surprise, confusion, often enlightenment. One of the most poignant was Gerald, who helped me for well over a year. He had been in the hospital more than ten years and was now in his late forties. He was rather odd and businesslike in his attitudes, seemingly always in a hurry. He occasionally made references to "atomic radiation" affecting him, and when pressed, insisted that a hospital doctor had done an operation on him, placing prisms on the sides of his eyes "to give me insight." Such was the logic of schizophrenia.

In spite of these difficulties, Gerald was an excellent helper, and I enjoyed being with him. In moments of lucidity he had a sense of humor and a generosity of spirit. His humor was difficult to recognize, because sometimes he meant the same comments one way and the next time another. His statement about prisms for insight was a delusion most of the time, but in moments of clarity, he thought it humorous.

When I left the hospital for another job Gerald went with me. He had been doing well enough to be considered for discharge. I needed someone to help me, and Gerald needed a job. A halfway house provided a protective environment in the evenings, and he worked for me during the days.

Gerald was blossoming, and I gave him gradually increased responsibilities. I was mindful of the hazards of transition after being incarcerated so long (I should have been, in view of my own difficulties in moving from a hospital to the "outside world") and I talked with him as much as possible.

I had to be away at some meetings for a week, and I asked Gerald if he would like to take a week's vacation while I was gone. He seemed pleased and agreed to it. I also alerted the halfway house that I would be away.

At the end of the week Gerald did not show up for work. I called the halfway house and was told he was in bed and would not come to the phone. I had a schedule of appointments, so Rita helped me that day at work. As soon as I finished, I went to the halfway house.

When I arrived Gerald was in bed, lying stiffly, staring at the ceiling. He looked awful. He did not seem to recognize me. He said he did not know me, and quietly added: "I'm dead." He had hardly eaten the whole week I was away, and he was weak and confused. Although the house manager tried to reason that since he could talk, he was alive, Gerald continued to insist that he was dead. I had been his lifeline, and when I went away it was cut, and he died.

I visited Gerald daily to try to reestablish our bond, but after a week the staff of the halfway house insisted he be returned to the hospital. I saw him there several times, but he wanted nothing to do with me. Although he was restored to the way he was before we met, he still refused to acknowledge that he ever knew me. When we had been together, he had begun to hope again for more in life, something he had lost in childhood. But the loss was too painful, and it was safer to feel and want nothing.

I had not realized how much our relationship had come to mean to him. Without my physical presence, he was "dead." This was not a metaphor, but a delusion. I felt devastated, almost as if I *had* killed him. The difference between us was that with Gerald, when I was out of sight I was gone forever, whereas I continue to remember him. Another lesson in relationships that I had to learn.

I was working eight to nine hours each day, and was on night call a couple of times a week. Not an excessive schedule for residents, but it taxed me to the limits of my endurance. I often exceeded my sitting tolerance, still only an hour or two at a time, and paid for it later in exhaustion. But I hated to ask someone to recline my wheelchair when it would interrupt proceedings, so I would tough it out, even though I'd often be numb to what I was doing. I was still trying to prove that I was as good as anyone. It was sheer vanity, because to everyone else the extent of my disability was obvious.

Rita would get me up in the morning; my attendant would take me to work and stay with me. Then in the evening I would return home and fall into bed exhausted, too tired to eat. I could not put such demands on myself today. But I had to overextend myself then, just to make it.

I longed to be able to do more things on my own. I could not wheel my chair, and being pushed always felt like being "pushed around." No one can ever move you exactly where you would like to go if you could do it yourself. No one can move you at the pace you would set for yourself, and no one can quite get you in the right position. In addition, helpful people often move you without asking you, assuming on their own that you would be better off in this or that position. Sometimes it is true, and sometimes it is not. Most times I would feel a mixture of gratitude and resentment.

An electric motorized wheelchair would be a partial answer, but none were commercially available at that time. I unsuccessfully tried to design and have one made several times. When at last a feasible commercial electric wheelchair was announced, I was the first to put in my order. Before it arrived, another very important event occurred in my life.

I had completed my training in psychiatry and my two years of supervised practice, so I was eligible for examination by the American Board of Psychiatry and Neurology. My new wheelchair arrived a few days before the examination. I was preoccupied with preparations for the exam, and I had prepared in my old wheelchair. I knew how I was going to do things from that position. It was familiar, even if I did not necessarily like things as they were.

Contemplating the exam and the new electric wheelchair together seemed like more of a strain than an opportunity. Even though I had waited long for both, I could only think about one at a time. Reluctantly I chose the exam, knowing it would soon be over. So I went for the examination in my old manual wheelchair, and was pushed around. It must have been the right thing to do, since I passed.

But when I returned home, free of the exam, the first thing I did was to get in my new electric wheelchair. It had a sensitive control that allowed me to operate it with a single finger. It was slow, awkward, and somewhat unreliable, but it was like being unshackled.

My freedom was largely illusory, since somebody still had to be with me to recline me. But it felt wonderful, like soaring. I do not imagine that an astronaut's lift-off at Cape Canaveral could have been any more exciting.

I learned, again, how dangerous it seems to take on something new, even if its advantages are obvious. Change is a complicated matter, whether for the good or the bad.

Change is continuous with the physical difficulties of a quadriplegic, giving life a feeling of instability. Nothing remains automatic or routine for very long. You cannot rely on your body to behave, so no sooner do you find a satisfactory way of doing something than it has to change. Then you have to find a different routine, or a different piece of equipment, so you are nearly always working to solve some problem or other—to find new respiratory equipment, corsets, wheelchairs, hoists, and mattresses to meet the current needs. Equipment failures are frequent and disrupting, for the equipment is unavailable while being repaired. Fortunately it is rare that everything breaks down at the same time, but there is always something. An old friend who has had polio about as long as I have dryly remarked once, "Sometimes I think if I had to do it over again, I just wouldn't get polio,"—as though he had a choice.

You do have to look hard to find any advantages in being crippled. There are a few. They seat you first on the airlines, but you pay for it later, when you get off last. There are "handicapped parking" places that are very convenient when some able-bodied person has not parked in them. Probably the one I appreciate most is at a Baltimore restaurant named Haussner's. The food is wonderful, and the service and decor are interesting. The main problem is its popularity. They do not take reservations, so there is almost always a long line waiting in front of the restaurant. The one exception is that they will seat you almost immediately if you are in a wheelchair, and they will, in addition, generously allow the people with you to enter at the same time. This has made me popular with friends in Baltimore. So far as I know, it is the only way to get into this great restaurant without waiting. There was a time when I felt guilty about such advantages, but there are so many disadvantages that the scales are overbalanced in the other direction.

But I have had my share of good luck. I certainly feel that way about my profession, and I have not found very many difficulties in working with patients due to my disability. There are the initial reactions, which anyone would have with someone who is severely disabled, but they quickly diminish as essential human qualities become primary. And people in need are usually just as willing to get help from a disabled doctor as from one who is not. Patients have enriched my life greatly. They taught me about aspects of life that I could not have conceived before, and in the therapeutic relationship—almost more than in any other—a deep level of understanding and intimacy is achieved. Of course, the expression of that depth is necessarily limited by the very clinical and ethical considerations that make it possible, and so also teaching the lessons of discipline and maturity. Most of my patients have generously given up symptoms of self-destructive behavior, grown and found good relationships, or whatever else they were looking for. This has further rewarded me, even though those relationships were reward enough in themselves.

When I finished my residency training in psychiatry, I was given the chance to be director of a new outpatient clinic at the hospital. In the course of developing that program I was brought into the mainstream of community life in important ways. I was forced to function outside of the cloistered security of a hospital environment, protected by the roles and rules of professions. I also had a little taste of power, and discovered how ambivalent I am about it. As an administrator I had to use my authority, but I never liked being a boss or being bossed around. I had to learn the difference between exercising legitimate authority and being authoritarian.

I was to have more opportunities. Within a year and a half I became the Director of Education and Research at the hospital, including the residency program from which I had so recently graduated. I still had to learn, and this was a marvelous opportunity, for if there is one sure way to learn something, it is to be required to teach it. That has been true for the things I have learned from disability, as well as the subject matter of psychiatry.

I felt a lot of compassion for the residents, and they became my friends and colleagues as well. In fact, some of them are still very good friends. There is a pleasure, not unlike that of participating in the growth and development of a patient, in working with the development of a psychiatrist. Some of the early lessons I learned from my patient/ helpers continued to allow me to move easily among the different roles of administrator, physician, teacher, and researcher.

I am pleased that one of the things that disability has allowed me to do is to see the human being behind the roles of patient, doctor, and others, and knowing a little bit about suffering and discomfort helps you to have some compassion for others.

One of the things that bothered me greatly about working in a hospital was that the patients' needs often had to fit into a narrow category of services, and the range of services was necessarily quite limited. Beginning the outpatient clinic was one means of providing greater continuity of care for patients. But a lot of other services were unavailable. I decided to design a plan to make the hospital a community mental health center, and for some time it became my major cause. I tried very hard to get it implemented against every kind of administrative obstacle, but in the end I was defeated.

5

Of Athletes and Cripples

No athlete is crowned but in the sweat of his brow.

—St. Jerome, Letter 14

I have lost all, but found myself.

—John Clark, *Paroemiologia*

A LTHOUGH the plans I had for a mental health center never came to fruition because of administrative obstacles, my efforts were rewarded in another way. The things I had written in my plan for the state hospital came to the attention of some administrative and academic leaders who liked the ideas. In response, I was offered a new position to develop and direct an educational and research center dealing with the social and community aspects of psychiatry. It was to be university-affiliated, with funds coming from both the state and the federal government.

The opportunity to create a new program and express my interest in the importance of social supports for people was very appealing. However, it also meant the disruption of the relative stability of our lives at the hospital. The choice was clearly between security and opportunity; between stability and risk. Rita supported me in choosing risk. There were many times when I had cause to doubt the wisdom of the choice, but in the end it was clearly the right one.

I was able to continue to see private patients and to teach as a medical school professor. This, along with some special research opportunities, made the package ideal for me.

It meant a new place to live, no longer the convenience of living on the hospital grounds. It meant finding new people to help me in my personal care, as well as recruiting for professionals at the Center. This was when Gerald, my patient/helper at the hospital, came to join me, as I have already described.

As director of the new Center I was given a new way of pursuing my old love affair with sports. The Center's mission was to study the relationship between social institutions and the development of mental health or illness. Sports are just such a social institution, and I could begin to study their effects on people—children, adults, and fans —with new resources and enough time.

As with most boys, sports were the single most important activity in my life when I was growing up. I fell asleep each night with fantasies of breaking into the foul circle to shoot a hook shot, leaping to catch a long pass in the end zone, or dashing away from the starting blocks on the track. In school, the education offered was little more than the price I had to pay in order to participate in sports. The important activities of school began when I left the classroom for the gym.

What I loved about sports was that they called into play all of my capabilities: power and guile, skill and discipline, force and subtlety. It was exciting to be able to use my body as well as my mind after the confined immobility of the classroom.

There are few activities in contemporary life that allow the full expression of mind and body. If a person works behind a desk, uses a computer or a typewriter, very little of his physical self is used. If a person works on an assembly line or in an outdoor job, there may be little mental challenge. Most jobs, including careers in sales, business, teaching, research, repair, or labor, require only a fragment of a person to be developed. Against a skilled opponent in an athletic contest you have to use all you've got, and more.

We live in a society that takes pride in being competitive. It is the "free enterprise" society, in which people are pitted against each other to prove their worth. Success is measured in achievement and money.

Sports and athletics have provided us with the vocabulary of the competitive free enterprise society. Winning and losing are the concepts which describe its activities, whether in politics, business, religion, or academics. We are advised to keep our "eye on the ball," and we admire a "good sport." We refer to presidents and other executives as "quarterbacks" and "coaches." To lower inflation, President Gerald Ford initiated a campaign called "WIN." If we work well with others, we are called "team players," and if somebody is knowledgeable, we say "he knows the score," and has "a lot on the ball." A person who acts inappropriately is called "off the wall" or "out in left field."

I was an athlete. I identified myself with all of the characteristics of that stereotype. I was strong and competitive, and I was a "good sport." I believed in fairness and playing within the rules, but most of all, I believed in winning. Losing was a sin, a crime, and a failure.

I was like a caricature of an athlete, so that when I became disabled, I even tried to turn my disability into a competitive sport. I did everything possible to deny the cripple in me. I had no use for him, and no place in my concept of myself for disability. Much of what I have written here has been about my search to find something of worth in that image of the cripple, something with which I could identify without regret.

At first glance the concepts of athlete and cripple seem antithetical. Although each describes an aspect of physical capacity and action, they represent polar opposites. Nevertheless, both require periods of serious training and retraining, and with both, performances are measured and records kept of how far one can go and how long it takes—the ability to manage in time and space.

But they are regarded very differently. The records of an athlete are a source of admiration; those of the cripple, a subject for pity. The former is calibrated in how much has been accomplished, and how "good" it is; the latter is seen as less than it should be, and how far there is to go.

Our society polarizes winners and losers, athletes and cripples, the successful and the failures. In a competitive society, victor is separated from vanquished by the "bot-

tom line," with athletes considered "better than" and cripples "worse than" the average.

My physical participation in sports ceased abruptly,
heightening my awareness of the effect of the loss on me.
However, even if physical ability does not cease so
abruptly, every athlete and every human being must face
and come to terms with declining energy, health, and ultimately death. And what every human being must learn is
that it is necessary to endure the hardships of life in order
to enjoy its rewards.

The athlete who insists he is a winner must deny his
disabilities and defeats. Yet they are inevitable parts of the
life cycle, as well as an athletic career. When he must retire
from sports because of age or injury, he feels like a loser, a
role he has been taught to avoid like the plague.

The neighborhood bars of nearly every city provide
testimony to how difficult it is for athletes to find meaning
in life when they have had to stop playing. How often one
encounters someone drowning his sorrows there, who
shows enthusiasm only when he speaks of his school or
college athletic career, when he caught a game-winning
pass or shot a crucial free throw. It is as though life stopped
with the end of the athletic career.

The doorman at the apartment house where I once lived
had such an empty life. The only time his face brightened
was when he told you about his days of glory, when he
pitched his third no-hit game in Little League. That event
had occurred when he was a child, but nothing that had
happened since was as important to him.

I longed to return to my cherished athlete/winner stereotype of myself. Nothing pleased me more than when I was visited by my old athletic friends and we would talk about the old days. Then I would deny what had happened to me and forget my new reality. However, I did ultimately have to go through the complicated process of mourning in order to look more realistically at athletes and sports.

I was lucky, for in addition to being a fan I was able to find a larger place in sports for myself. As a psychiatrist, I began to see athletes as patients, and later I was a consultant to individuals, teams, and major professional sports organizations.

An old friend helped in a surprising way. She was publisher of the largest tennis magazine, and desiring to be helpful, invited me to write for it. I became the book reviewer, since I could not attend tournaments as they were happening. I wrote scathing criticisms of a number of tennis books, unconsciously expressing my grief and rage over my lost involvement as a player. I was a spurned lover who hated the love I could no longer possess. I raged against innocent writers telling athletes how to become winners. The reviews were so negative that my friend frequently had to ask me to tone them down.

Later, when I was able to get around in a wheelchair, I covered a couple of important tennis tournaments for the magazine. I was still in the process of mourning, though, and neither the winners nor the losers escaped my acidulous comments about the play. It was an important cathartic expression for me, and helped me to begin to recognize that losers were as human as winners. I fear this unusually public process of mourning did not help the circulation of my friend's magazine. But I am happy to say the magazine survived and flourished in spite of my writing.

It was important therapy for me, and I no longer felt so deprived afterward. Though I was not able to compete on the field, I had become involved in other aspects of the game. Had there been no way for me to return to sports, the abruptness of the termination of my athletic career might have influenced me to continue to idolize the pre-disability part of my life, recalling only the best parts.

I might have continued to think of myself as *only* a winner before polio and *only* a loser afterward. Having another opportunity in sports allowed me to correct idealization with information and reality. Viewing sports from different perspectives opened my awareness to broader meanings and brought their importance down to scale. It brought the role of the athlete into more nearly correct proportions, neither bigger nor smaller than life.

When my grief and anger had dissipated, I could see sports from a more neutral position, neither a lover nor a hater. Then my criticism became more refined. As a somewhat detached but interested observer, I began to see things that I had overlooked about the way athletes and teams participate, and I began to recognize how different styles affected winning and losing. I began to understand the importance of coaches, administrators, and especially fans.

Much of what I observed athletes doing did not seem

goal-directed. I noticed that for many athletes elaborate rituals seemed necessary for them to focus their aggression.

Hitters in baseball must knock imaginary dirt from their spikes, spit on the ground, and dig in before they are ready. Basketball players bounce the ball a particular way and repeat certain motions before shooting a foul shot. Tennis players make seemingly meaningless gestures before serving.

It is a rare athlete whose physical capabilities can be directly expressed without some kind of ritual, and the style of play represents a unique integration of the winner and loser images within them. If effective, the style allows a place for every aspect of the personality of the individual and the team.

The path to victory would not be so tortuous if these images of winner and loser, athlete and cripple, did not exist within each athlete. Most identify only with the athlete/winner and try to avoid recognition of the loser and cripple within them, so they function as incomplete people. Inevitably we are all both winners and losers, and we must find ways of valuing each aspect of ourselves in order to use our full potential.

When one part of a person is avoided, denied, or alienated, it tends to return in hidden ways—ways which disturb the person's equilibrium and interrupt his goal-directed behavior. We can find out something about those interferences by noticing the expressions, gestures, and styles of players.

Some athletes seem able to win only if they come from

behind, while others are front-runners and must hold the lead from the beginning in order to win. Some continually berate themselves for errors during the play; others try to find a way to blame opponents. Some excel under pressure, and others "choke." Some play best when angry and when they feel cheated; others are upset and do not play well at all in a hostile environment. Some prefer the crowd to be with them, and some do best when it is against them. Some are best as team players supporting others, and some are best as soloists. Many are complex amalgams of these extremes, and how they behave at any moment depends on the context. Although physical factors may influence these styles, the psychological ingredients often are even more significant.

When one team defeats another or one athlete beats another, the words used to describe the event betray some of the underlying meanings that create problems. We hear that one player "murdered" another, or a particular team "annihilated" the other. The losers were "torn apart" by the winners, or "it was slaughter." We hear the fans shout encouragement with words such as "Kill 'em" or "Take no prisoners."

These are not terms which accurately describe a sport or play, even a competitive sport. The rules have been established specifically to protect the participants against injury and support the play in a civilized manner. However, that these descriptions are commonplace implies how they are perceived, with the words representing the unconscious significance of the play—what is hidden beneath the veneer of rules and roles of civilization.

While the rules are designed to protect the players from injury, they and the fans are attracted to the possibility of violence. Violence does sometimes erupt when the players become mindlessly engaged in the play, forgetting the difference between playing within the rules and "maiming" their opponents. They may even seek to injure them.

For the participants in the play of competitive sports, the unconscious significance is that of a life-and-death drama. The winner is the murderer with blood on his hands, and from that standpoint he must atone for his guilt. The loser has been killed or maimed. The concepts of the loser and the cripple remind athletes of their vulnerability and mortality. Within these meanings of the contest, the athlete uses rituals of style to ward off danger and guilt.

Insistence that we are *only* athletes and *only* winners is the effort to deny the inexorable effects of the forces of nature. If we do not allow ourselves to think that we are mortal and deny our disabilities, we think we can keep them away. The athlete plays as children play in an effort to retain that youthful denial. It is a vain attempt to drink from the fountain of youth.

A ranking tennis professional was once one of my patients. He was troubled by his inability to win long matches. He had a power game, and if he could get his big serve in the court and make decisive volleys, he was able to quickly dispatch his opponents. When he could do that, he remained untroubled.

However, if a match became extended and developed into a long, grueling struggle, his play gradually deteriorated, until he lost. So he lost to many players of inferior skill, and it was well known among them that if they could keep him on the court for an extended period, he could be beaten.

During those long and arduous matches he noticed that he became very preoccupied with his health and his capacity to survive the physical strain of the match. Every minor ache or pain became a symbol of some fatal illness. He also, curiously, had similar concerns about the health and safety of his opponents. He worried when they became fatigued, and got agitated if he observed them develop a limp or some other physical evidence of disability. He was in the habit of quickly dismissing these marginal thoughts and feelings because they seemed so irrational to him, until he began to examine them in psychotherapy.

As we considered the problem he was reminded of his father, who had suffered from a chronic disease and had an agonizingly slow death. This recalled even earlier memories, when his father seemed extremely powerful and he, a young child, had enjoyed wrestling matches with him. Then, as he grew older, he was appalled watching his once-powerful father waste away.

As a child he could express his full competitive desires without fear of being harmed by his father, and there was no danger of his harming the man himself. His father's strength had served as a protection against the full force of the child's aggressiveness. Then, as he saw his father decline and become vulnerable, he realized this man could defend neither his son nor himself against attack. The memory of a crippled father losing his battle against disease returned to haunt his sense of himself as an athlete and winner whenever he was involved in a long, hard match. Then it seemed like a matter of life and death, rather than a tennis game.

The long match reminded him of his father's long decline, and it laid bare the vulnerability he experienced and sometimes attributed to his opponent. Without an internalized protective father, the "killer instinct" aspect of competition was exposed. Winning and losing long matches held the implications of murder and torture for him. It was only in the mercifully quick match that he was safe from the emergence of his worst fears.

Another patient was a major league baseball player whose career was failing because of a curious restraint he felt about throwing the ball. He was a catcher with a "good arm," but his ability to throw to the bases became severely compromised and he was unable to throw runners out. His throwing inhibition gradually worsened until he actually had difficulty just returning the ball to the pitcher. At that point he was put on the disabled list.

He'd grown up in poverty because his father was unable to hold a job and worked only intermittently. His father had an explosive temper, and even as a child he often was in the position of protecting his mother from the man. He hated his father's capricious authoritarianism and despised his lack of success.

As soon as he was able, he left home and left the memory of his father behind as well. He began to prepare himself for a major league baseball career with great intensity. As he approached the realization of his ambition, the success he dreamed of, he could no longer isolate himself from the nearly forgotten image of his father. Success required, in his mind, the annihilation of his father, but the loser image and the failure he associated with his father were only apparently forgotten, and at the pinnacle of success these images returned. He had forgotten the guilt he felt about leaving his failed father and vulnerable mother behind, and now, when success was in reach, it returned. He could not allow himself to succeed without finding an acceptable place for his father within him.

As he became more accepting of his memories of his father, he no longer had to separate that part of himself. It was not the stereotyped loser that he had to accept, but the human qualities of losers that he had denied. He had been terrified of the appearance of the loser in him, and in trying to blot it from his mind he was obliterating a part of his potential strength. Coming to terms with the associated terror and rage was necessary for him to regain his ability. Then he could return to baseball.

A college pole vaulter reached record-breaking heights during practice. However, in competitive track meets his performance was only mediocre. Practice was play for him, and in play he could fully express his capacity.

Competition, however, represented something serious and real for him, and in real life people can get hurt if they let themselves go and express their aggressions fully. He viewed defeating an opponent as though he were doing bodily injury to him, rather than simply achieving a higher standard on the pole. The pole vault symbolized life-and-death issues, not simply athletic competition.

His mother and his grandmother had died within a year of each other when he was quite young. They were the two people to whom he was closest. Both were very protective of him, and like most children he had entertained aggressive fantasies expressing omnipotent childhood wishes for freedom. When these two important people died, he erroneously assumed that his wishes, and sometimes his "bad" behavior with them, had been responsible. Defeats of opponents in the pole vault were like flashbacks to childhood, when he believed his wishes could come true, and he was responsible for them. To beat an opponent was to kill him.

As he learned more about the cripple and loser fantasies within him, he discovered that they were alive and resilient. He realized that losing and disability were not final states, but rather aspects of all human life.

All of us distort reality by seeing it through the lens of past experience. The athletes I have described viewed athletic contests as though ruled by the law of the jungle. Each one distorted reality in his own particular way, and turned athletic competition into a field where the winners survived while the losers were maimed or dead.

No winner is ever permanent; no athlete is perpetually strong and healthy. Success is only momentary, and in the next competition he may be beaten. And even if he wins frequently, ultimately he will be beaten by others.

The cripple stereotype represents the wounded warrior who has been not only defeated but rendered helpless, unable to defend himself in the unconscious world of atavistic struggle against death. That stereotype symbolizes the fear of all future defeats, and the ultimate one. In reality, the cripple is impaired only in some ways, unable to do only certain things. He is not disabled in every way. He may be a winner in many other ways.

The person who can find no place in his life for the loser must deny aspects of his own humanity and the humanity of others. He is ill prepared for the vicissitudes of everyday existence and the difficulties within the life span. We are all athletes. We are all winners at times. We are all cripples at times, and ultimately we all lose to death. We must be open to every aspect of who we are in order to be able to respond appropriately to the changing contexts that develop in life.

But what is the alternative? What is there of worth to be found in the images of loser and of cripple? What can be learned from them that can become valuable? What are the redeeming qualities that need to be integrated in a person's concept of self?

If losing is not seen as a permanent condition, part of a larger process, a person can learn much from defeat. He or she can learn forbearance and discipline, the ability to endure and to take the bitter with the sweet, as well as what must be done in order to win the next time.

Of Athletes and Cripples · 91

The ancient archetype of the cripple shows how complex the image really is. Vulcan, the crippled Olympian god, was also among the most physically powerful, showing that strength and weakness exist in the same person. The idea that wisdom develops out of hardship is shown in the cripple as magician, possessing knowledge not revealed to others.

Disability separates the cripple from conventional habits and places him outside of the average and normal. As an outsider he can see much that is obscured to the insider—the inevitability of loss, defeat, and disability, things that allow a person to roll with the punches and to acquire value from each experience.

There is much to be learned from the experience of defeat and the role of cripple, including the old-fashioned idea that by "meeting your responsibilities" you do something worthwhile, regardless of victory or defeat. This allows people to endure difficulty and live satisfying lives under arduous conditions. There is success in doing your best even if it is in the process of defeat, and defeat in a "good cause" may well be better than winning for a bad one.

If a person believes that the universe begins and ends with his individual success or failure, he is utterly and totally alone, a prisoner in his narrowness. By accepting that the loser is in each of us, we learn something important about the meaning of life—that it is not limited to the successes and failures of any one individual, but that together we all are part of the sweep of evolution.

6

Flying Without Wings

No bird soars too high if he soars with his own wings.

—William Blake

SEVERAL YEARS AGO, I saw a small bird hopping about in search of food outside the window on the lawn. Its movements seemed awkward. It had to jump from place to place, as though its legs were bound. It had no arms or hands to reach with, so it had to bob up and down with its head to poke about the ground for food. That bird and I were kindred spirits. We both had bound legs, useless arms and hands, and were forced to grub about just to survive. We were deprived of more meaningful and fulfilling actions.

Then quite suddenly the bird unfolded its wings and rose quickly off the ground. It banked sharply and soared high above the trees. It was all grace and power now, and not a trace of awkwardness remained. It climbed higher and higher, until I had to strain to see it at all. At last it disappeared from sight, but while I watched, I realized my spirits too had risen.

Folded wings and bound legs make the bird a prisoner in time and space while on the ground. Opened out, they become a way to soar; for what is useless in the lowest plane may provide access to the highest. Reality comes in many forms, and can be used to bind or free. That bird had the same wings on the ground and in flight, but had put them to very different use. Perhaps I could use what happened to me for a different purpose too.

Some people seek and accept the very things that I hated and fought against in my disability. The religious faithful seek salvation through fasting and deprive themselves of worldly pleasures. Hindu worshippers voluntarily endure pain from sharpened spikes on beds of nails to achieve higher consciousness. Ascetic monks stand motionless for hours at a time. They simulate the tortures of the flesh endured by their saviour on the cross as a means of purifying themselves. Pandit Nehru said the strength and wisdom he showed in later life came from learning to use his time in prison well. These people had enriched their lives by the same physical restrictions and limitations that I felt demeaned by. Was it also possible for me to achieve some higher purpose by my suffering?

Those people who willingly endure suffering similar to mine do so because they have a purpose for it, a cause that is served by their agony. My problem was that I could see no special value in my suffering. I longed for such a purpose—one to which I could fully commit myself and for which I would be willing to endure anything. Like "good old Charlie Brown," who said that when he grew up he would like to become a "fanatic," I would happily sacrifice myself to such a cause.

The last time I could remember being willing to die for

something was during World War II. Virtue seemed on our side, and you could tell the good guys from the bad guys. But if there was one thing that everyone should have learned from that period, it was to be wary of causes, and that the most heinous crimes in history were committed against people in the service of what from one standpoint was a good cause. That tempered my full commitment to traditional political movements and orthodox religions. I could see virtues in nearly all of them, but when implemented too literally, they could not be trusted. I have become involved in various movements since World War II, but always mindful of the lesson of the Nuremberg Trials—that I, not the movement, am responsible for what I do.

But that did not keep me from longing for something to die for. So I had recurrent fantasies of a suicide mission for some great, unspecified purpose. A thinking human being was required to carry it out, but physical ability was irrelevant. An honorable death seemed far better than the life I feared. But what an irony that I should need something to die for to make living worthwhile.

My purpose in living had to fit me, and I had to begin by making explicit what my purpose in living was. Even if it did not form a coherent ideology, I had to identify some individual ideas that held strong value for me. I had to create my own cause.

The first thing I realized about myself was that I needed to live with intensity. Since childhood it had been important for me to do whatever I did well. While that was a start for me, it still did not identify my purpose and *what* I was trying to do.

I remembered a principle that I had learned in medical school: the "Primum Non Nocere," which means "First, Do No Harm." And I knew that was important to me. I did not wish to harm anyone. I first thought with some irony that, indeed, that philosophy was aided by my physical disability, for it was unlikely that I was physically going to hurt anyone while lying on my back.

But, of course, there are other ways that I could hurt people, and besides, there was a more positive way of considering the issue—that I did not wish to do harm because people, and all life, are valuable. Albert Schweitzer's concept of a "reverence for life" was something I could embrace. I thought of it, perhaps more narrowly, as attempting to find the integrity and worth in everyone and everything that I encountered.

Discovering the worth and integrity of others was a natural extension of a great curiosity I had always had to see the world from other people's viewpoints. I was filled with wonder whenever I would grasp how different my interpretations of events were from someone else's. This would make me realize that I was a part of a grand design, far larger than I could comprehend, and it was like a religious experience.

That supported my sense of myself too. If every living thing has value, I am included, and my thoughts and feelings have some worth. Although many psychologists believe the development of personal self-esteem is necessary *before* one can recognize the value in others, it seems to work the other way as well to me. When I can appreciate what is unique in others, I feel better about myself.

Although I did not understand it clearly at the time, I have come to realize that my beliefs are also those expressed in Martin Buber's concept of "the I and the Thou." What I now understand Buber to mean is the capacity to experience another person subjectively, from the inside, as though you were actually him or her.

When you look at people as objects, all you see is the surface. They are things which could just as well be inanimate; moreover, there is little need to know details, for you simply see the same thing again and again, and to recognize a category is not to know an individual. There is only tedium and deadness in a category like ceiling, iron lung, or person, unless what is unique, changing, and special becomes apparent. That's how I wanted to see everything—as a living, changing subject. To see something in that way you have to be able to identify with it, to be able to imagine what it would be to be in that position, and to be able to see more than just the name of a person or a thing. It means studying what it would be like from the inside, and not assuming immediately that you know what it's like just because you recognize the surface appearance.

Frequently, when we notice things it is because some change has taken place; that is, there is some action which hits us. But also, it is possible to make active changes in our focus of perception by taking something from the background in our field of vision and bringing it to the forefront. Then you perceive a different picture.

Take, for example, those popular pictures in which with one focus you see a beautiful woman but with another you see a leering skull. The focus changes as you switch the background into the foreground, and vice versa. You can play in the same way with whatever you see, hear, feel, taste, or smell.

The principal things in my environment looked like the same old room, the same ceiling, the same iron lung, even the same people who took care of me. But I began to realize that these things are never really the same, but are always changing—the moods, the light, the color, the context, and what has come before—all transform from moment to moment. With each of these changes outside of me I am changed, if only I allow myself to be affected. I had to look at each of these moments in space as though it were a new one.

I had moments of great pleasure and satisfaction when I became absorbed in observing minor details and becoming an *active* observer, rather than a passive one. Not only sensory pleasure, although that was certainly a part of it, but the pleasure of creation, of living creatively, of establishing a life in the face of whatever adversity there was. The capacity to see everyone and everything from an alternative view, most especially from the standpoint of the other person or thing itself, enlivened me.

I realized this had happened on that night when the

depressing hallway turned into an artistic creation of dark and light shadows.

I began to think of the purpose I sought in living life artistically, seeing the world with an artist's eye. These were no longer abstract concepts for me. Rather, they personified the ideas of Schweitzer and Buber, the "reverence for life," and "the I and the Thou."

I finally knew what I wanted to be when I grew up. I wanted to be someone who had reverence for life, who saw others and even other things as subjects, Thous, rather than objects. I wanted to be an artist, creatively living my life. This was not a cause to die for; it was more important —a cause to live by.

Eventually, I could pass a very interesting time looking at the ceiling, noticing small details and changes. I could also see it as if it were the floor. Then the overhead light fixtures seemed to stand upright, and the chairs and tables hung from the ceiling. I played with the sounds I heard, listening now to the voice tones of a speaker, and then to the words, then perhaps shifting to some background noise in the room. Instead of looking only at people's eyes I noticed noses, and ears, and mouth expressions, and skin color. I began to see others in ways I had not seen before, in richer ways.

I saw color in place of form, and vice versa. I found I could eat colors, instead of the tastes and textures of food. I had memorable virtuoso experiences, like the day I saw people's shoes as dramatized expressions of their owners' innermost feelings, saying, "I'm run down," or "I don't fit here," or "Aren't I cute?" Or when I realized I could hear birds singing in some whirring machine noises.

Sometimes I could even do it with pain and other forms of severe discomfort. I would not fight the feelings, but would embrace them fully, as though I had chosen them. I could then begin to feel their pleasure, and surprising things often happened. At the very least I was not bothered as much by the pain.

Sometimes, if I were lucky, I would become like a child and perceive the world like an ever-changing kaleidoscope picture.

Whatever happened, this kind of experimentation—artistic living, as I came to think of it—gave my life a sense of freshness in place of tedium. Even though I could not move, I could actively engage with whatever was around me through the play of my senses. I was no longer entirely dependent on movements in the environment; I had a purpose and a means of action. I could be more than a helpless victim, and I could have a part in determining my life and what shape it took. It was an important step toward feeling like a human being again. My wings felt like they were beginning to open.

7

Not Enough

For Sale: one used tombstone. Splendid opportunity for family named Dingle.

—Madison (Wis.) *Capitol Times*

WHEN LIFE fits our expectations, we think of it as an opportunity. When it does not, we think the *world* failed us, not our expectations. But that is a mistake, for life will be whatever it wants to be, and not necessarily what we want.

There are many diseases and disabilities of the body, but there is only one plague of the mind. It is to believe that one's life is not enough.

When I became disabled, and my life changed so dramatically, I could not believe it, and I hated it. I thought of myself as healthy, strong, and vigorous. I wondered, "Why did this happen to me?" I thought I was exempt from such things. Other people may have been destined for illness and disability, but I wasn't one of them. I thought I knew who and what I was. Strong and able, I could not possibly be a cripple! I would not have it.

There were some other curious things that made what happened to me especially hard to believe. Two major determinants of susceptibility to polio are exposure to the virus and fatigue. More than a year before I contracted polio, I had worked in a hospital during a polio epidemic, and was constantly exposed to the virus, as well as excessively fatigued by twelve- to fourteen-hour days. I assumed that if I were ever to get polio, that would have been the time. Instead, it was over a year later; I hadn't been exposed to the virus as far as I knew, and I was not exhausted from working long hours.

The Korean War began during the last few days of my internship. When I was alerted by my Naval Reserve Office to prepare for my induction as a medical officer, rather than continue for just a few weeks in my residency or begin a practice, this seemed like an opportunity to do something that I had always wanted to do, which was to play in the major national and international tennis tournaments. The timing was perfect. The close of my internship also signaled the beginning of these tournaments. I planned to play until I was called to active duty. In what at the time seemed like great good fortune, the Navy did not actually call me for four months.

That four-month period was very special to me. It was as though everything good was happening. First, I had completed my professional training, and for the first time did not have to think about that grind. Medical school had been very demanding. In order to make ends meet, I had—in addition to my studies—held down various jobs all through medical school. I was always pressed for time, short of sleep, and under great stress. My internship had been almost as bad, with long hours and high stress.

But during that four-month period before I was called

to active duty there was no work to speak of, no sleep deprivation, and the only stress was that of tournament play. My physical condition was better than it had been for many years, good enough so that I was ranked among the top twenty. I had not seen a case of polio for well over a year, and I was living under the most luxurious circumstances of my life at the resorts and clubs where the tournaments were held.

Then it happened. For some reason the virus found a hospitable environment in my body. In a matter of hours I went from feeling strong and agile to being barely able to stand, unable to stand at all, eventually unable to move, and finally not able to breathe.

There is evidence that there can be stress when too many good things happen at once. However, I certainly did not experience my newfound freedom as stressful, as far as I can recall. Quite the opposite. I can remember writing home about how wonderful life seemed. So in my sickbed I wondered, "Does it mean that if things are good, you have to pay for them? Is good fortune inevitably followed by bad fortune?"

My belief was that the universe was an orderly place, and there were cause-and-effect relationships that determined all things. I also believed that there was justice in everything. Good deeds were rewarded, and bad ones punished. Perhaps my illness was some form of justice. Perhaps I had done some terrible thing.

I searched my memory to recall what crime I had committed that would merit this punishment. I was obsessed with trying to find that fatal flaw. Was it when I talked back to my parents? When I was unpleasant to my blind date? Or . . . oh yes, it must have been the day I carelessly lost my brother's sweater! These things were all that I could think of that might be the source of my misfortune. As I write this I am embarrassed that I did not have any worse crimes to remember. However, at the time my conscience made them seem possible sources of what had happened. Now, less confused and hopefully clearerminded, I find them not only human but too absurdly mild, considering the exuberance of youth.

It now seems to me that mine was but a child's belief in an orderly world of justice. I now think that if there is order in the universe, how the system works and what produces what is well beyond the comprehension of human beings. Why one person is affected and not another cannot be answered by men. Why something happens now and not at another time is beyond our understanding. And what form the justice of the universe takes is not something we can use.

I desperately wanted to find some logical explanation. I even considered the concept of Karma. It is an orderly belief system about the universe, and a way of finding explanations and justice for whatever happens. Since there may not be an *apparent* rational basis for whatever happens, it postulates that one is punished for what happened in past lives. From this point of view I must have committed some terrible crime in a past life, and punishment in the form of disease and disability in this life served the cause of universal justice. But I think it is more likely that such a belief was just another childish attempt to bring order out of apparent chaos.

I can well understand the need for that, because when I first became disabled and my body failed me, one thing that had not changed was my beliefs. I certainly did not want to have them destroyed along with my good health.

Even though I could not find a convenient cause-and-effect relationship for what had happened to me, I was heartened to realize I still could learn from the experience. It *does* make sense to me that one tends to find himself in situations that he can learn from. Life is unpredictable. Whatever ways a person limits himself by thoughts of how life should be, he probably will face realities that are in conflict with those limits. There must have been something to be learned, for my disability has been a very persistent teacher.

When I began to learn from my experience, one of the things that I had to face about myself was a form of greed. Specifically, I had wanted to sample everything. I wanted to travel everywhere and see everything in the world. I wanted to meet every kind of person and know all about people. I wanted to know all about everything. I felt as though if I had not seen it, I did not know it, and if I had not done it, I was missing something. I had been constantly in search of a variety of experiences, knowledge, travel, and all things. Even my eating habits were symbolic of this greedy perspective. Although I never ate large quantities of food, I did have an insatiable desire to try every variety of cuisine.

There is not anything particularly wrong with this attitude in itself, but it has limitations. That is the lesson I needed to learn. Knowing something about everything is not the same as knowing one thing in great depth. Tasting every experience does not produce the same effect as savoring a single experience. I was an effective taster, but I soon looked to the next adventure. What I had needed to learn was how to take and accept one thing, one experience, and to find the adventure in that one. Disability stopped my search for variety, so I had to come to terms with what *was* available to me. In the beginning it seemed *not enough*. I wanted more.

Comparisons were a big part of the problem. I compared my present state with how I had been before. I compared my inactivity with the many things I used to do. I compared my weakness with my former strength. I compared my current situation with my childhood aspirations. Comparisons. I realized that is how I had been living my life. And most of the comparisons were invidious. I was not doing as well as I had been, as my friends and colleagues were doing and I *should* be doing. My life was not enough for me.

Comparing myself with others at one time may have been very useful in spurring me on to improve. But now it mainly produced a sense of despair. I could not be as I wanted to be, and I could not do what I wanted to do.

Perhaps all of these comparisons were really only shadows of more subtle influences: my parents' aspirations for me, what I had learned in commercials on radio and television, what I saw in movies and in books and newspapers. These were all stories of the strong, the virtuous, and the handsome, and of their good deeds with the just rewards that followed. But I had been removed from the "Pepsi generation," and I could no longer be the "Marlboro man." The Brylcream look was an impossibility.

I had had a stepladder view of life, behaving as if it were my task to keep climbing ever higher, trying to reach some mythical pinnacle. Now it seemed that not only was I several steps down from where I had been but I had fallen all the way to the ground.

Eventually I began to realize that the stepladder had assisted me well, but now I needed to acquire a new perspective, one that would serve me in the current situation. Very dimly at first, I began to accept that life has ups and downs, like a roller coaster—some predictable, some not. There are moments of excitement, of relative calm, of fear, of pleasure, and of danger. On a roller coaster, it is fun only if you go with each experience and allow yourself to discover all there is in it. If you are set against the experience, the most you can hope for is survival, and you will miss the richness of the ups and downs.

A few years ago I heard a sick joke. It seemed to fit my situation. It was that "death is nature's way of telling you to slow down." Although perhaps less pungent, disability was nature's way of telling me to slow down. I had worked toward trying to improve myself and to make things as I thought they should be. In order to do that I needed to know all the possibilities, so I kept looking for new ones. Now I had to learn to live in the present and to discover a way to live with, and hopefully even enjoy, the very limited options which were available to me. I had to discover how to make the most of what came my way, rather than making things happen by my activity.

I realized that there is a choice of attitude, of perspectives on life. You can look at situations for what is missing, how they can be improved, and what ought to be. But you can also look at them this way: that this is the only time and the only thing available, and it cannot be compared with anything else in the world. The choice is between the agony of not enough and the excitement of adventure.

In health I had approached the world from the standpoint of perfectibility. I could always be improved, and the world could always be improved. I had a keen eye for flaws wherever they existed, and I had developed certain skills to eliminate them. I was the stereotypical housewife so preoccupied with discovering dirt that she has no opportunity to enjoy the fruits of her labor. The person who, looking into the clear, starry sky, only compares it with what he saw last night will miss the wonder of the universe. My task was clear—to extend the dimensions of my interest in what could be seen *now*. What became new and exciting was this idea: that perhaps the power to determine how I looked upon life was within me. Whether I considered my disability a great tragedy and a loss or whether I saw it in some more positive light might just possibly be a matter of my discretion. If this was true, and it seemed increasingly likely that it was, new worlds of belief and perception were open to me, and new hope for what my life could be was waiting.

The concept that the glass can be seen as either half empty or half full is hardly a new addition to the wisdom of the ages. But to see its application to my disability, where I could find only limited possibilities for change before, seemed very special. And anyway, the things which I discovered that are profound and important to me always turn out to be the things that I already know.

8

The Choice

It is often simply from want of the creative spirit that we do not go to the full extent of suffering. And the most terrible reality brings us, with our suffering, the joy of a great discovery, because it merely gives a new and clear form to what we have long been ruminating without suspecting it.

—Marcel Proust

TWO COMMANDOS penetrated deeply into a hostile country on a highly dangerous sabotage mission. They were captured by an army patrol and immediately brought before a firing squad. They were bound in chains and surrounded by a thousand soldiers with automatic rifles poised. The command was shouted: "Ready, aim . . ." At this point one of the doomed commandos turned to his partner and whispered, "I've got a plan."

That is the way I treated my illness, as though there must be some way out of this mess. My disability was a problem to be solved. It did not occur to me that it could not be worked out, and that my persistence in trying was a delusion of power in one so blinded by fear that he could not accept reality and surrender gracefully to it.

I had grown up with the belief that if someone wanted something badly enough he could have it, and if you were willing to work hard enough for something, you could always get it. These beliefs came both from my parents and from the period in history in which I grew up—the first half of the twentieth century. The pioneer spirit seemed to fit the realities of that period.

There were real advantages to harboring those values, for it promoted optimism and well-being. It also produced self-fulfilling prophecy. The fervent belief that you could make something happen often led to such strenuous efforts that it actually did.

The country had not yet encountered its limits. In the pre-nuclear age we believed that if you were right and strong, you had a power over destiny. We had not met adversaries who were just as strong and as certain that they were right. We thought all problems were soluble by improved technology. We had not yet seriously polluted the oceans and the rivers, and had not yet depleted the land.

I personally was no more prepared for facing an insurmountable problem than the country was, for I was its product. I wanted to change what had happened to me with every fiber of my being, and I spent long hours for many years dreaming, scheming, and planning ways in which I might return to full function.

As far as working "hard enough," I do not believe that anyone could have worked harder at his rehabilitation. In fact, that effort became a detriment in several ways. Patients were told that the degree of improvement would be equal to how hard we tried. We did not know then that beyond a certain point exhaustion produced even further damage. We were told that the enemy was the contracture that developed in the weakened muscles, and that we must endure pain in being stretched. I was so willing to endure my share, that I have several muscle groups that have been seriously overstretched.

So firm was belief in hard work among the people I encountered in rehabilitation medicine that nothing would dissuade them. If you were not improving the way you hoped, it was simply, in their view, that "you didn't want it enough." Perhaps they were not so rigid as I remember, but rather it was the stricture of my beliefs at the time that I was dealing with.

If I were to give up my cherished conviction in being able to make things better, I would have a void in my belief system, and I did not have anything to replace it. I did not have some way of regarding my life which would allow me to live with it. Surrender seemed a matter of cowardice, and I did not want any of that.

Only as the years wore on and forced me to realize that my limitations remained unchanged did I begin to consider alternatives. I felt as though I were dragged, kicking and screaming, toward this new version of reality.

"God give us the grace to accept with serenity the things that cannot be changed, courage to change the things which should be changed, and the wisdom to distinguish the one from the other." Reinhold Niebuhr wrote this "Serenity Prayer" in 1943. Perhaps there were lots of other people at that time who had trouble accepting things that could not be changed, and perhaps they had difficulty too in distinguishing between what could be changed and what could not. The wisdom to choose between what should be struggled against and what should be accepted is at the heart of the problem, and there is no formula to solve that in a rational way. It only comes when the time is right, and when certain work has been done.

My task involved two processes that occur simultaneously. The first is giving up the old and the obsolete, preparing the ground for something new. The second is having something positive that is available for a new commitment.

The first process, dealing with loss, is one that is fairly well understood, and has been described by many writers, of whom Elizabeth Kübler-Ross is best known. It is the grieving process, and involves a gradual reduction in the investment of energy committed to something or someone who has been lost. The stages described are the same whether it is for the loss of a loved one through death, the loss of a community through moving, the loss of a physical function, or the loss of an ideal.

The stages begin with denial, the insistence that one has not lost what is valued. Then comes blaming, trying to find someone, something that caused it to vent one's rage on. When this fails, there is bargaining; bargaining with a doctor, with God, with the universe, that if I do this, will you give me back what I have lost? Then, when one discovers that there is no one else to blame or bargain with, no one to rage against, despair and depression appear. And then we are told that there is acceptance, and this is where the misunderstanding begins.

The question is, acceptance of what? We are told that it is acceptance of the loss, but why would anyone be willing to accept the loss of something valued or loved unless he had something of nearly equal worth to embrace? The more important acceptance is not the reality of what has been lost, but the acceptance of something new that is valuable and can take the place of the loss. Without something new, one clings to the past, for the fantasy is more palatable than the present. If one discovers that there is indeed nothing to replace it, there is no further reason to go on. Many people who perish during periods of loss and transition do so not because they have not accepted the reality of the loss, but because they had nothing to replace it.

When I could find no one to blame, and when the bargains were not struck, I was alone with myself in my despair, my loss, my depression. But these things in themselves did not lead me to acceptance of my disability.

For there had to be a positive replacement. During that initial period I spent my time trying to be (as much as possible) as I had been before. But the more I associated myself with the past, the more I was aware of how things had changed. The more time I spent in familiar circumstances, the more I was aware that they were unfamiliar and unrewarding.

Some things were helpful transitions, things that would allow me to find a new way of being, involving old enthusiasms. The first and most meaningful was sports.

Then, perhaps most important, there were the people in my life—a few close friends and family members who did not give up on me. But even with them my role had to change, and in some cases the change was not mutually satisfying and the relationships ended.

In addition, I did with some friends what many people who become disabled do—I avoided them. I did not want to have them see me and know me in this new way. It seemed too humiliating, so I cut off the relationships. This was especially true with young women for whom I had cared and who had cared for me.

And finally there was work, a job that I could see for myself. Although I could not be a surgeon, I could see a profession that I would value, and a place where I would have a useful and acknowledged position. But that took a long time.

9

Acceptance

The common problem, yours, mine, everyone's
Is—not to fancy what were fair in life
Provided it could be,—but, finding first
What may be, then find how to make it fair
Up to our means.

—Robert Browning

GIVING UP the old attachments and giving up the emotional charge that binds you to the past involves the stages of grief. I had to stop clinging to an obsolete image of myself as an athlete, as an able-bodied person, as a particular kind of lover, as a traveler, and so on. Reducing my commitment to those obsolete images in itself did not provide me with something to accept, but only with a void where there had been something, like soil waiting for a new seed to be planted.

Often it is at this stage that a choice of whether to live or die is made; whether to give up or to go on. Among my friends who were in rehabilitation centers with me, some chose to die, not able to see any meaningful life. Others, unable for some reason to die physically, had a living death instead.

The man on my right in the rehabilitation center died when he could not see a replacement for the life he had as a telephone lineman, and he could not see a new relationship with his wife. The man on my left had the support of his family, but he could not accept a new role in the family.

So he went home and for twenty years stayed in the same room, in the same bed, until mercifully he finally did die.

My competitiveness was useful in keeping me alive, and I found a new way of living in the hospital, so that my emotional life looked promising. But I realized that even more might be possible. I was out of the iron lung in my wheelchair during much of the day, with enough energy to consider other things—things that would allow me to support myself and live as other people did. I certainly did not want to be institutionalized for the rest of my life, but to avoid it I had to find some new activities I could accept and a different lifestyle than I was accustomed to. And again I had to enter uncharted waters.

In order to accept something new there must be time, there must be fertile soil for growth, and there must be an adequate replacement that can develop. Only if these characteristics are present can graceful acceptance occur with dignity. Otherwise there is only emptiness and humiliation.

The stages of acceptance which need to occur simultaneously with the stages of grief are as follows:

1. Rejection of the unfamiliar options.
2. Looking for something new.
3. A grudging acceptance of something new.
4. Behaving as if you accept it.
5. Discovering some of the same satisfaction in the new that you had with the obsolete.

6. Surrendering with dignity and grace, or embracing the new as if you had chosen it.

During the stage of rejection I would not even consider any alternative to the way I had lived and who I had been. If someone were to try to encourage me or even make a suggestion, I would reject it out of hand. It seemed as though I was being offered crumbs when I had been used to eating a full meal. My friend on the left in the rehabilitation center would make such rejections with wry comments such as "Yes, I've always wanted a tin cup with pencils."

As the futility of this rejection out of hand began to wear thin, I began consciously to look for things that might be enjoyable and meaningful. At this stage I would "try on" different things in my fantasy, and, where possible, in reality. A simple but important example for me had to do with baseball. It had been my least favorite sport, for I had grown up in Southern California when there were no major league baseball teams there. Yet throughout a large part of the year, baseball was the only sport heard on the radio and, later, seen on television.

I had to make a deliberate effort to find something of interest in baseball, and to do so as a fan, not as a player. It was hard, but as I understood more and more about the game, it became more meaningful and satisfying.

Similarly, I had to consider what a love relationship might be like for me, and I did this quite consciously. I was very fortunate in that even though I had rejected the relationships I had before as being impossible, I began to meet people who also seemed to care for me. That made it seem possible to have new friendships. Gradually I was able carefully, inch by inch, to test out how acceptable I was. When I got support, it gave me courage to think about what marriage and a sexual relationship might be like with my disability.

Then I began to think also about work opportunities. My first choices had to be rejected as I learned more about them and what they demanded. But in the end one choice seemed possible: I could see myself as a psychiatrist, although my early thoughts about what it involved now seem bizarre.

Behaving as if you accept involves two things. The first is trying out in fantasy what it would be to be the person you envision. This is an extension of the previous stage. The second part is actually beginning to engage in the tasks. For me it meant actually becoming a sports fan, acting as if I were one; it meant learning enough about psychiatrists so I could act as if I were one, and beginning to date a woman as if I knew how to under these new conditions.

At this stage it is especially useful to have a model, someone who has suffered your loss and done the same things you want to do. For me it would have been to know sports fans and to know how they behaved. It would be knowing a disabled psychiatrist and how he might behave, and knowing someone who is disabled and how he might behave in a love relationship. Unfortunately I could find very few models, so I really had to find my own way for the most part. Today it would be easier to find models in one of the many independent living centers for disabled people. Here one is apt to find people who work, people who are married, and people who have a variety of avocations while still being severely disabled. There are also more disabled people who have become integrated into society and are visible today.

I was largely on my own, and without models. So I was probably more cautious in exploring options than I might have been had I known others who had covered the same ground. The fear of appearing foolish and of being rejected caused me to be timid. I learned by trial and error.

Almost everything has the potential for embarrassment under new conditions. Risks are not easily taken if the consequence of failure is to feel entirely alone. Ultimately it is left to the individual to take the risk. This may mean simply closing your eyes and jumping blindly into it.

I vividly remember the first time I went to a public park, the first time I rolled down a public street, the first time I ate out in a restaurant, and the first time I went to a movie. These seemingly small risks loomed very large at the time.

The encouragement of family and friends can be helpful, but it is also limited in value. People who have known you before you were disabled tend to talk about the "good old days." That was one of the problems I had with my old tennis friends. When we got together, that was all we spoke about. Although I enjoyed those fond memories of the past, they had a destructive relation to the current reality. I needed a better way of becoming the new person who was taking shape inside my mind.

Support groups for people with disabilities can be very helpful by offering models and opportunities for sharing experiences. Unfortunately many disabled people find it hard to use these groups. They have the same stereotyped concepts of disability that normal people do, and so do not want to join a group known by its weaknesses. To do so seems like giving up and joining the losers. Of course, what one actually learns from such a group is that people do not behave like stereotypes. Quite the opposite. Each person is supported in his uniqueness.

Each time I tried something new I was afraid of failing. And I often did. Then I retreated until I felt enough support to try again. Sometimes the support came from the encouragement of others and sometimes from inside, when I would screw up my courage to take the risks.

I had to reconstruct a new life from damaged and rusting materials. It required new skills in relationships, work, and recreation, new means of mobility, communication, and expression, as well as polishing up the old ones that remained intact. I will describe how this happened in the next chapter, but here I want to emphasize the stages of acceptance common to all risks.

Sometimes the steps I took were too large for me to handle. Then even if I got away with it, and adequately went through the expected motions, I was only halfway there. It is much better to take one step at a time than to make a grand leap.

It is not easy. Inevitably there must be awkwardness as one learns to accept that new personal needs and desires are legitimate, even when they are out of the ordinary. The same sense of fullness, joy, and absorption are possible. This is critical, for hope that is not nourished by reality soon dies. One needs to recognize that there is indeed something of value in the new existence, something that will not suffer by comparison with the old.

Acceptance with dignity is surrender without a sense of capitulation. One lives *as if* he had freely chosen the new life. It is a stage when one enjoys the new opportunities for their uniqueness alone, savoring them as full and total. In this period grace comes from the fact that the disability has been integrated into a new way of life. Any awkwardness which occurred in the earlier stages now dissipates. Life as it is is "all right," and experienced as good, or as it should be.

Self-acceptance is not something that occurs all at once or, for that matter, once and for all. It is a very gradual process that comes in tiny increments, so small that they are not usually noticed. I often realize that I have accepted something only afterward, when I compare how I feel now with how I had felt before in the same situation.

For example, I used to feel crushed and humiliated when I needed help from someone and they did not want to do it. I would blame either myself or them. But the sting I felt has now diminished. Getting help for my needs is more of a business transaction, and I no longer feel like I have to act like "the brave little soldier." The change also became evident to me when I could interview prospective personal-care attendants and discuss their duties without embarrassment.

Still, there is deep within me the feeling that I am a tiresome burden to the people who help me and, as a result, I am often compulsively apologetic about my needs. This is the most stubborn area of my self-rejection, but I notice even this is changing in subtle ways.

Perhaps these descriptions may sound as though I am unnecessarily touchy and self-effacing. However, I have found that it is an unusual disabled person who has not had similar feelings. Self-acceptance is a lifelong struggle for me and, I believe, for many other people.

This recognition allows another level of transcendence —one that is paradoxical, and so beyond any simple concept. A person experiences himself as both unique and ordinary at the same time. Separateness links us to all others. We can see the world through our eyes alone, yet we know somehow that there must be a larger vision that envelops all of us together. It is a state when life is experienced not as an obligation but as a gift, an opportunity alone.

These stages are not necessarily either final or complete. I find that my relationship with my disability is similar to a marriage. We have an agreement, my disability and I. It requires that I take care of it, and it will allow me to do what I want—it will take care of me. It is not an altogether unfriendly relationship. Sometimes it is even a love relationship. Sometimes it is the relationship of a teacher and a student. My disability has taught me much, and continues to do so. It teaches me about limitations and about the hazards of pride and vanity.

Frequently, I see my disability—no, let me restate that —I *prefer* to see my disability as an adversary, an opponent or an enemy to be overcome and battled with. This is very useful for me sometimes, and allows me to try to compete against it, to try to beat it, and gives me a clear focus for my effort. It is interesting that when I think of my disability as an enemy, it is a male adversary. I try to face him squarely, to look him in the eye, and to hold my ground. I have to deal with my fear so I can see my opponent clearly. I have to challenge my enemy and beat him at his own game. I must know and be able to acknowledge when I am helpless before him and there is no alternative but to surrender. I cannot be deceived by the power that I feel at one moment or by the control he exerts at the next. That power is only experienced in relationship to my adversary, and sometimes our relationship changes.

When I accept my fear, I accept and respect the power of my opponent, and he no longer dominates me. We join together.

When I do surrender, my disability becomes female, and we are united in that special way that men and women can unite. We are in confluence, and the relationship is perfect. We are in agreement.

If I abuse my disability or ignore or reject it, it will

defeat me. I must pay attention to it, but I cannot give it my full attention lest it become my obsession. My disability is relentless. At times we are separate, and at other times we are totally absorbed together. We can never be totally divorced, but we can live separate lives as I go about my business as though I were not disabled. At these moments my disability is nowhere in my awareness, and it has no significance at all in what is happening. But what I must do is be continually open to its messages, because I know that if I ignore it completely, it may, at some time, take over completely.

This is especially true with regard to my energy, which is very limited. Sometimes I can get away with overdoing things a bit, but if I stay up a little too long or do not have quite enough respiratory support, I will have to pay in the end.

There was a time when I used to think of myself as a prisoner in an iron maiden. My disabled body was the iron maiden, and I was the prisoner within. In that medieval torture machine, my disability encased me fully, even as I struggled against it. But when we have become one and I identify with it, it becomes me and I become it. I realize that the iron maiden becomes my handmaiden and a pleasurable companion.

To fight or to surrender, to try to make it better, or to take reality as it is—the choice is still there. But where does Reinhold Niebuhr's wisdom to distinguish one from the other come from? It must come from a place we are not used to looking—from a place that can be discovered only by letting go and stepping back. It is a place that appears only in this moment that you cannot plan for, but can only be open to.

To accept gracefully something that is awful seems impossible, and a contradiction in terms. But once you get the hang of experiencing things from the inside, anything becomes possible. The changes are so gradual and subtle that they are difficult to define. Surrender and acceptance are talents which must be learned.

So I have learned a great deal about acceptance as well as fighting back, and it has helped me to understand a lot about myself and the nature of being human. Still, there is the question about how I will regard things in the future.

When I was young and physically strong, to live life from a wheelchair was unthinkable. When I became disabled it was unacceptable, but gradually, over the years, not only did it become acceptable, but I found it satisfying as well. Now, at those times when even the freedom I have in my wheelchair is threatened, I wonder if there is anything that is really unacceptable from the subjective standpoint. Or if, on the other hand, I will not be willing to accept most things.

When I contemplate life without my wheelchair, when I can no longer do some work and have contact with others who have meaning for me, it is frightening. When I think of living in a situation where my only contact with others would be as a patient to their care-giver roles and when there is no substantial hope of improving the situation, it seems like the ultimate horror story. I would not be able to accept it now. But sooner or later I know that I will face something again that seems horrible to me. Will I once again gracefully find a way to accept what now seems unacceptable, or should I be prepared to take what measures I can to end my life before I have to face them? The choice is between the way of Socrates and the way of Jesus.

Jesus went to the cross and gracefully accepted the horrors of crucifixion. Socrates, when given the choice of living without his major purpose and meaning in life, teaching, chose to die. Would Jesus have chosen the quick certainty of hemlock over crucifixion if the choice had been offered him?

There is still the question of whether to try to accept whatever comes to me, to acknowledge "God's will," or to take matters into my own hands and exercise my will. If I am to seek to live an existence in God's image and have my will coincide with his, there can be no master and no slave. There can be no other to whom I surrender my autonomy. There is instead only one godlike pathway, but it is one which I cannot anticipate until it emerges in the moment.

There are practical implications for society. One man survives because a hundred doctors and nurses and technicians using millions of dollars in medical equipment keep him alive. A thousand children die because they do not have the most elemental resources to feed them. The man who is kept alive artificially may have no purpose larger than his own survival, miserable as it may be. Would it not be more life-affirming for him to call a halt to the use of those resources to maintain his misery in favor of helping a thousand others to survive?

When I think about the choice between fighting and giving in, and of its ultimate application with regard to life and survival, the matter becomes complicated. But then I recall that the correct choice, the God choice, will emerge at that moment, and not before. And then I remember the lesson I must learn over and over again, that the specific applications of true wisdom are not yet written, and will emerge in time. I then feel relieved. The dilemma seems to dissipate. I have to remember to look with fresh eyes at this moment, and open myself to what is before me without prejudgment and without a preconceived plan.

10

Humor and Enlightenment

MASTER: What are you doing?
STUDENT: Nothing.
MASTER: How will you know when you are finished?

NOT LONG after I became disabled there was a week when everything went wrong. Besides my own disability and helplessness, I learned that my brother had a fatal illness. Then a few days later my stepfather suffered a stroke, and my mother, the last healthy member of the immediate family, got the flu. I was desperately worried about my family and frustrated by my uselessness to them, and, of course, they could not help me either. It could not have been worse, I thought.

Then the irony of the situation came to mind, and I began to laugh. I doubt that I could have satisfactorily explained the joke to anyone else, but it was a godsend when I saw it. The reality had not changed, but I felt better.

A person can cry only so long without the tears beginning to develop a life of their own. Eventually sadness and tears offer a spurious security by themselves, with the world viewed continuously from a down position. But humor and the laughter it brings allowed me to emerge from despair into the light of day. For a moment I could see with clear eyes again, and that allowed for a fresh start. Humor can be a way of mastering a situation that seems otherwise to have no solution. For me it has been a source of support equal to medical and nursing care—something that made illness and disability not only bearable but at times enjoyable.

When I could recognize something funny in what a moment before had seemed like a hopelessly grim situation, a wonderful transformation occurred. It was as though I had been suddenly healed and restored to health, even if only for a moment, and even if only in my mind.

I still feel relief and my sense of well-being is restored whenever I can laugh or find something to smile about. It gives me a new perspective on life; what an instant before seemed insurmountable and tragic becomes quite acceptable. For now, at least, things are okay. It is as though my mind, my body, and my spirit coalesce again into a unified whole and my place in the universe is restored.

The salutary effects of humor not only are internal but also influence relationships between people. Humor and its unique expression—laughter—are more contagious than the common cold. Anyone with direct contact is likely to get it too. Then it is difficult to feel estranged from someone with whom you have laughed.

I remember once arguing furiously with someone with whom I worked. It was obvious to me that it was folly to do it any way but mine. He seemed to believe the same about his way. Then in a moment of passion my energy was spent, and I could not make a sound. I just did not have enough air, so I had to stop, and then I began to laugh. I saw some obscure irony in my blustering without air. Suddenly he began to laugh, and we were no longer adversaries, but were in that moment together.

Although in such situations the facts of the unresolvable conflict have not been changed, the shared experience of laughter causes adversaries to rise above pettiness. As with a flock of birds that have been foraging for food on the ground, when one lifts its wings to rise, the others follow to the higher plane. There is an unmistakable conflict-free closeness that occurs when people share laughter, just as it appears when birds are in flight. Perhaps both are reflexes designed to show us that we are not alone.

With humor not only do I feel more whole inside, and not only do I feel closer to those about me, but I also feel a quality of elevation, raising the realm of consciousness to a space that is larger than before.

Laughter is something from the gods, and it sets us on an Olympian plane, where we are no longer the victims of mean circumstances. We become integrated into some larger perspective. It is a perspective that nurtures us back to health for a moment, and restores aspects of ourselves which we thought we had lost forever.

Humor and laughter are so commonplace that people tend to dismiss their full significance. Since humor and laughter are rarely very far from any situation and can emerge at any time, we tend to overlook what they can do for us. We are like Dorothy in *The Wizard of Oz,* who in the end discovered that what she was looking for over the rainbow had all the time been in her own backyard.

There is an expression, "funny as a crutch," which is used to suggest that there are some things that are so tragic that there is no room for humor. To say that there is nothing funny about a crutch may seem obvious; however, I can assure you that for those people who use crutches there is much they find that is funny about them. Wherever disabled people congregate, whether on a hospital ward or in an independent living group, or simply when friends gather together, there is an "in" humor that deals exactly with the frustrations and predicaments of being disabled. Though these things may seem tragic or shocking at the time, and certainly would appear so to the nondisabled, they may have a very different effect on those who have spent their lives with disability. They have learned that, like any other aspect of life, there is an underside of wheelchairs, braces, crutches, and other appliances which can be seen as humorous.

A group of my friends, who were patients at the rehabilitation hospital when I was there, get together frequently. We are all still disabled. There are many things we found humorous then, and still laugh about now on occasion. The day that Lyle became so angry at a fellow patient that he tried to take a swing at him, even though he was unable to rise from his bed. The day that Andy became trapped in midair, in a patient transport device, and the attendant could not get him down. Then there was the time when a paralyzed patient was floating in the swimming pool supported by an inner tube which gradually lost its air. The look of utter despair on his face as he slowly began to sink below the surface now creates gales of laughter when it is recalled (of course, he was rescued). There are scores of such instances which in their own context we experience as hilarious.

Once Rita and I went to lunch at a lovely beach restaurant which was perched high on a hill overlooking the Pacific Ocean. It had only a small flat area near the entry where lifting me in and out of the car was possible. After our enjoyable lunch Rita left me in the flat area at the top of the hill while she went for the car down below in the parking area.

The entry was not as level as it seemed, and the brakes on my chair did not hold. Slowly I began to roll down the hill, creeping at first, gradually picking up speed, and before I could call for help I was well on the way down. The seconds that followed seemed to extend for a long time, and they are sharply etched in my memory. I was helpless to do anything about my predicament, and I was heading for disaster.

Once the inevitable was established, a feeling of peaceful surrender engulfed me. So I actually enjoyed the last few moments. I felt like I was a downhill skier, completely enjoying the exhilaration of movement. Unfortunately my enjoyment was abruptly interrupted when I collided with the side of a new sports car.

The impact was absorbed by my right leg, and I immediately started to go into shock. I was pretty sure it was broken. Rita and a busboy, who had helplessly witnessed the whole event, reached me in a few moments. They got me to lie flat in our car to counteract the shock, and we left for the nearest hospital.

But as we drove off, steam began to rise from the radiator and the temperature gauge rose off the scale. Realizing that she could not drive further, Rita pulled in at the first store to call the paramedics. They promptly arrived and efficiently whisked me off to the hospital. I persuaded Rita to stay with the car to get it repaired while I went to the hospital to get my own repairs.

By the time I got to see the doctor, I was recovering from the shock. I told him what had happened, explained my symptoms, and said that I thought my leg was broken. He made a cursory examination and agreed that it was "probably broken." Then, glancing at my chart, he said, "Oh, I see you're a psychiatrist." He did not wait for a response, but continued: "I've been having a lot of trouble with my weight, and I seem to be getting heavier and heavier. I've been wondering if it's really because I'm depressed. Do you think I should take an antidepressant drug?"

Still feeling considerable pain, I mumbled something to the effect that it was difficult for me to consider that question since I was preoccupied with my broken leg.

But undaunted, he continued: "What do you think about taking an antidepressant drug as a way of losing weight?" Again, trying to put him off, I said something

146 · *Flying Without Wings*

about not feeling like talking about it because my leg hurt so much.

He continued: "If I were to take an antidepressant, which one would you recommend, and at what dose?"

Well, from the accident, I had learned something about surrendering to the inevitable, and clearly this guy was not going to give up. So I mentioned the name of the first antidepressant drug that came to mind and told him a standard dosage. This seemed to please him, and he smiled, telling me, "Well, I think we better get an X ray now, to make sure about your leg."

As he walked away, I felt stunned and couldn't believe what had just happened. Then the absurdity of it struck me, and I began to laugh. Soon I had completely forgotten about the pain.

A little while later the doctor returned, holding an X-ray film. He held it up to the light so I too could see, pointed to an area, and said, "Yup, it's broken." Then he continued: "I've really enjoyed talking with you, and got a lot out of it. I'd like to come to your office and see you. There are some other things I'd like to talk about."

Hardly believing what I heard, I reminded him that I still had a broken leg and did not know how soon I would be practicing again. I added that, besides, it was difficult for me to think about it under the current circumstances. I told him I was sure he could find a competent psychiatrist nearby, so he would not have to travel so far to see me.

But he was nothing if not persistent. "No," he said, "I have a relationship with you, and I know I can get more out of talking with you." Remembering what I had learned about not fighting what is inevitable, I simply agreed, but I could not help smiling to myself.

Fortunately, by that time Rita had arrived at the hospital. Since I had no working musculature in my legs that would pull the bones out of alignment, the fracture itself was no problem. A simple soft cast could easily hold it in place.

A team of nurses and orderlies got me into a rented car, and Rita and I were off for home. The last thing I remember as we pulled out of the hospital yard was seeing the doctor cheerfully waving goodbye. I never heard from him again. Perhaps the antidepressant drug had actually worked; then again, perhaps another psychiatrist had unsuspectingly wandered into his emergency room as a patient.

Tragedy and comedy certainly are both impostors. If you look at one very closely, you are likely to find the other.

By the next day my pain had subsided, and having survived, I was in inappropriately good spirits. Every few minutes I would remember the amusing events with the doctor the day before, and I found myself chuckling.

I was able to get an orthopedist to come to the house to confirm that I was doing the right thing for my leg. He was a sober man who thoughtfully examined me and confirmed that we were handling it correctly.

Because of my curiously punchy state of cheerfulness, I

remembered an old joke. So in my intoxicated state I playfully asked the doctor, "When my leg heals, will I be able to walk?" The poor man, not knowing the extent of my paralysis, was a perfect foil, and gravely answered, "Yes." I could hardly contain myself, and it was only between chuckles that I could deliver the punch line: "That's wonderful. I couldn't walk before."

He did not smile. He did not laugh. In fact, what I had said did not even seem to register as remotely funny. His seriousness only made me laugh harder. I'm sure he was convinced that my problem was less in my leg than in my head.

On a ward full of disabled people, gloom can sometimes descend in a heavy cloud. Each patient feels uniquely victimized. This was especially true for those of us who got polio in the 1950s, for it was only a couple of years later that a vaccine became available. As a result, polio has all but disappeared.

Just after I left the hospital, I received an advertisement sent out to physicians by a pharmaceutical company promoting its polio vaccine. The cover was a magnificent color photograph taken with an electron microscope of the polio virus, blown up so that it was the size of an earthworm.

I managed to get a dozen or so copies of the picture from the pharmaceutical company, and made them into Christmas cards for my fellow polio victims. My wife was concerned about how they might be received, and it was very interesting.

All of the former patients found the cards hilarious, and enthusiastically thanked me for them. But my wife had insight into the feelings of the patients' family members. Many of them could see only the tragedy of the situation, and they either ignored or were incensed by the picture. The victims, however, could see the irony and humor. They had lived with the tragedy so long that they welcomed a way out.

The able-bodied person is likely to be appalled by "disabled humor" and find nothing funny at all about it. But it is like a man slipping on a banana peel. It is funny in one context and tragic in another.

Humor about disabilities shares much with "ethnic humor," "black humor," "army humor," and "gallows humor." All of these deal with desperate circumstances—the ultimate tragedies—discrimination, death, illness, cruelty, and the like, all of which do lend themselves to humor and laughter.

Some young friends told me about their mother's death. She was a wonderful woman who died heroically after a long, painful, and eroding cancer. The family spent as much time with her as possible, and felt the tragedy of her suffering and impending death deeply. One day, when she was quite close to dying, she opened her eyes to speak. They leaned close to hear what might be her final words to them. She whispered, "Who killed J.R.?" (referring to the popular television show Dallas). The family members having expected some profound deathbed statement, began to laugh. The woman, who had not laughed in many weeks, joined with them in what is now recalled as a beautiful final moment together.

At the funeral, missing her terribly, they were each alone in their sorrow. The pall over the family members who had lost their mother was deep and heavy. Then the priest called upon those who wished to speak about the deceased. The first to arise was the neighborhood busybody with a long prepared speech about her "dearest friend." The whole family knew she was only a distant acquaintance. Their initial shock turned to a shared amusement that lightened the service and restored the family members to the spirit of their mother, who also would have seen the humor in it.

Humor may reveal the relationship between victim and perpetrator, equalizing their respective positions. One of the experiences that are often most difficult for the disabled is when they are patients on a ward and become an unwilling audience for "holier than thou" evangelists who condescendingly come to "elevate their unfortunate souls." Often religious zealots fervently believe that illness is punishment for sin and that the disabled are "sinners."

Once a particularly offensive evangelist came to our ward, berating us for our sins but insisting that if we were to repent, the Lord would provide whatever we asked. A seriously ill and rather confused patient blurted out, "I need a bedpan," stopping the unprepared evangelist in his tracks. He had no intention of being of practical assistance, and after a couple of embarrassed mumblings he fled from the ward to gales of laughter from the other patients. For a moment reality had been given a twist, and the victims were restored to equal power with the able-bodied.

There were many people who visited our hospital wards out of religious conviction, and the vast majority were kind and generous as well as well-meaning. The few who were offensive unfortunately had colored the way those of us on the men's ward viewed all of them, and they did not deserve it. We displayed arrogance at its worst by making them the butt of our jokes, and this proved you do not have to be able-bodied to be arrogant and pompous.

One Easter Sunday my friend in the next bed groaned aloud to warn me: "Look out, here come the evangelists." I could see them across the ward, walking from bed to bed, pausing briefly to say something, then moving on. They carried a basket of paper flowers, each with a biblical message on it. My friend's warning and my own prejudice made me want to avoid them. So when they came close to my bed I feigned sleep, an easy matter since I was already lying motionless on my back, with my hands crossed on my chest.

A man and a woman, dressed in the uniforms of their order, came alongside my bed. They paused and looked at me. One turned to the other and said, "Let's not wake him. He looks so peaceful; we can leave him our message." They carefully selected a paper flower and message from the basket. Then they paused to look for a suitable place to leave it. Spotting my hands on my chest, they gently wove the stem between my fingers so the flower would stand upright. I lay there like a corpse holding a last flower as my two morticians slipped silently away.

The whole ward had watched what had happened, and began to roar with laughter. The tables had quite innocently been turned on me, and I had received my comeuppance.

I had taken it upon myself to assume a superior position to those I feared would act superior to me, but once again the roles were equalized. I had inadvertently left myself open to ridicule. I had planned to trick those good folk and belittle them for their faith. But the cosmic humorist alone knew who was making fun of whom. It was poetic justice.

Humor is a great equalizer, elevating the victim to the level of the perpetrator, diminishing the self-inflated, and showing the kinship among people. It also shows that tragedy and comedy are but two aspects of what is real, and whether we see the tragic or the humorous is a matter of perspective.

Of course, there are moments that are beyond humor, and for that matter, beyond tears. When there is no other side to the situation for the person experiencing it, he can only react. Holocaust victims tell me that after days of thirst they were so weakened and desperate they could think only about clinging to life. I have been with fellow patients so preoccupied with the next breath and whether or not it will come that they have no energy for laughter or for tears. And there may be humor on the way to the gallows, but not in the hanging itself.

At these times the humor and the desperateness are so extreme that individuals are reduced to automatic, almost subhuman responses, mindless reactions which are probably not greatly different from those of any animal in such a tragic state.

And humor and laughter may sometimes be used for a nefarious purpose—not to equalize and to rise above, but to belittle and to make fun of, to put down. Humor is man-made, and so can be used for whatever purposes men have.

There are many things that must be taken seriously, and to make jokes about them is a means of diminishing their gravity. Here, humor becomes a cop-out, a way of salving one's guilty conscience for not taking a human stand. This applies especially to those situations where it is possible to change the reality. For example, I find little that is humorous in the jokes about nuclear war, because nuclear war would be a man-instigated, man-made horror and thus one which human beings are in a position to influence. I prefer not to diminish the intensity of the need to face the consequences of such a disaster by laughing about it. I have felt that way about many things.

But for the person faced with a situation where tragedy is an accomplished fact with an inevitability about it, seeing the humor in the tragedy allows a way out by discovering a larger picture. Thereby a person discovers more of the potential that resides within him. One of the heroic things about humanity is its phoenixlike talent to rise from the ashes and take flight again.

John Stuart Mill long ago observed that every concept is true in one perspective and false in another. Humor reveals the same thing, showing that ideas by themselves can easily be transposed incorrectly. Recognition of different perspectives is an essential characteristic of humor and one that opens the choices available for people to see more widely.

Getting trapped in a narrow view of life has a deadening effect on a person and on those he tries to influence. The worst crimes in history have been perpetrated by people with good ideas which they stretched and warped beyond their context. Laughter, and humor that promotes it, restores the context and opens the eyes and ears more fully to the magnificence and the beauty of living.

The here and now is the only place to witness this richness and its many possibilities. That moment is known by many names—the holy instant, the moment of peace, the eye of the hurricane, the moment of completeness, wholeness, and health.

Yet, ironically, the moment cannot be frozen, but must move in a fluid and continuous way as we move on. The alternative of being caught, out of context, in an earlier time, in an earlier place, causes one to miss the possibilities and potentialities that forever arise. Openness is required for a full life.

In order to maintain a continuous sense of peace, one must be continuously changing. There is apparent conflict between having clear vision and sticking to firm beliefs. But the kaleidoscope of life must be open and selective. It is one of the fundamental uses of humor to restore the flux, therefore balancing tragedy and comedy, victim and perpetrator, life and death. We must be willing to see the humor in what we take seriously, but equally willing to take seriously what we laugh about.

I have found one uniquely personal irony: because those muscles which would allow me to breathe are paralyzed, when I laugh I do so without making a sound. I have the internal experience of silent laughter; my face and body motions reflect that I am laughing, but no sound is emitted. Since I value humor and have found it a wise teacher and an agreeable companion, it has special meaning for me. It reminds me that the sound of spoken words does not necessarily reflect the experience within, and what is manifest may be a shield to conceal the truth. Similarly, to experience the fullness of life it is *not* necessary to articulate it in traditional ways, and this realization has made me less dependent on conventions.

I sometimes think of my disability as a Roshi, a little Zen master, who is always with me, enigmatically smiling at my struggles. His task is to teach me the meaning of life, but he does this by indirection, never telling me clearly what something means. He benignly confronts me with the absurdity and contradictions in the way I look at things. Like all good Roshis, he is apt to strike me when I become complacent, and if I ask too many questions, he will counter with a question.

My Roshi also makes use of koans, those paradoxical statements and questions which make it impossible for me to depend solely on reason or principle, no matter how elegant it may be.

If taken too literally, a koan produces frustration and despair. Consider this example, one of the most familiar of all koans: "What is the sound of one hand clapping?" When you try to explain the unexplainable, you cannot. Then you are forced to give up your narrow and literal beliefs. Out of the confusion can emerge a truth beyond words and stories, one that casts the individual into a higher plane of consciousness.

Just as I think of my disability as a Zen master, I often find a koan in humor and jokes about disability: "Is there laughter without sound?" is one example. It is a realistic question for me. The question is a metaphor for the larger, more important ones: "Are peace, happiness, and joy possible if one is severely disabled?" A koan cannot simply be answered in words any more than the experience of disability can be easily conveyed. A Zen student seeks to find an alternative. The koan is an invitation, not an explicit statement, but one that helps to show that there is more to life than what is confined by description.

Zen masters also use stories as guides for the student. For example:

Two Zen monks on a pilgrimage came to the banks of a swiftly moving river. There, a young woman stood fearfully, unable to cross. One of the monks immediately swept her up in his arms without a word and carried her across as he and his companion forded the river. He set her on the opposite bank and continued his journey without a backward look. After a time the other monk could stand it no longer and admonished his companion: "You know you are forbidden to touch a woman, yet you carried that woman across the river." The first monk turned blandly to his companion and responded: "I set her down at the edge of the river. Are you still carrying her?"

Some of my experiences have become my Zen stories. Once at a party I was introduced to a vivacious young woman who seemed quite taken by me. She felt compelled to tell me all about her life and did her best to find out about mine. We were talking at the edge of the dance floor, but my voice was too weak to be heard above the loud music playing in the background. As we talked, she had to lean ever closer to my face in order to hear.

But as she closed in on me, she leaned into contact with the electric control which drives my electric wheelchair. Unknowingly, she began to drive my chair forward in fits and starts. She was so engrossed in the conversation that she was oblivious to our movement and unconsciously maintained her closeness to me by artful footwork.

Out onto the dance floor we moved, lurching this way and that, to a rhythm never played before. Although I tried to explain what was happening to her so she would stop, she could not hear me. I thought to try to take control with my own hand, but my efforts were blocked. The control switch appeared to be lodged waist high in her skirt, just at the level of her genitals. My fear of getting caught while making an obscene pass was greater than my growing terror about the outcome of our movements across the dance floor.

We continued to move among the dancing couples; she remained oblivious to what was happening; and I continued to be inhibited by what might appear as a sexual overture. At last we collided with a stunned couple, pinning them against the opposite wall. My companion, never hearing me, continued to talk and ask questions as though nothing had happened.

The memory of that dilemma is a Zen story worth remembering—one that can be relied upon to expand anyone's consciousness of disability. Best of all, it is a story that makes me laugh now as much as it did on that first occasion.

Zen students frequently laugh at the moment of enlightenment. It expresses the experience of relief at sudden contact with reality. If a student reaches satori—that continuous state of enlightenment—he will maintain the feeling state that approximates the burst of laughter, a state of open-mindedness and wonder. It is what a child must feel when he is suddenly surrounded by playthings, unencumbered and free.

Nearly all jokes are populated by the images of disability and the strong, and nearly all have the potential of revealing some hidden truth about each:

DRUNK: "Pardon me, what time is it?"
MAN WITH WATCH: "Ten o'clock."

DRUNK: "I must be going crazy. Every time I ask somebody, they tell me a different time."

The drunk, disabled by alcohol, sees something more clearly than the man with the watch, who embodies conventional strength.

The qualities of space can be illuminated by a joke as much as by a great work of art.

To honor his wife, a wealthy businessman, ignorant of art, commissioned a portrait of her by Picasso. He engaged Picasso at great expense because he understood him to be the greatest painter alive at the time. When the painting was unveiled, the businessman was outraged, for it was a typical Picasso representation, filled with his own idiosyncratic expressions. Angrily the businessman confronted the artist: "This doesn't even look like her!" Then, taking a snapshot of his wife from his wallet, he thrust it at Picasso, saying, "Here, this is what she looks like." Picasso calmly took the little picture, studied it for a time, then blandly turned to the businessman and said, "My, she's very small."

If time and space can be perceived in so many different ways, can we ever be entrapped in them, or are we not free?

I like to think that koans and Zen stories, which are accorded such a lofty place by many, are not much different from American jokes and humor in their effects. The power to reveal reality is in each.

An important part of any joke is the punch line, but the punch line is meaningless without the buildup of the story.

The story by itself is simply a statement, and perhaps not even a very interesting one. The punch line by itself is meaningless, and if you start with it not knowing the story, the humor is lost.

We all know the outcome of life—the punch line: sooner or later each of us must die. That is the punch line that equalizes everything. But people who are prematurely focused on death and try to just get it over with are vastly mistaken. They actually know *nothing* without knowing the process of what goes before the outcome. There is no humor or laughter in the outcome alone, and there is no wisdom in the story alone. You have to go through the whole process of the joke to know what it is.

Humor and jokes, and perhaps even koans and Zen stories, are like churches and religions. They can be used to elevate humankind and to seek that which is holy and godlike; or they can be used for purposes of self-justification and cruelty.

As for me, humor has more than comforted me through some difficult times. It has helped make sense and meaning of my disability. Even common everyday jokes have shown me the profound in the mundane, and the complex in the simple. That makes tragedy fuse with comedy, and helps me to find my place as a part of the universe, while I stand apart from it.

11

Antaeus and the Paradox of Change

open your thighs to fate and (if you can
withholding nothing) World, conceive
 a man.

—e. e. cummings

THE ANCIENT Greek myths have always held a special appeal for me. These stories of the Olympian gods and heroes seem to relate directly to essentially human qualities, and expose naked desires and feelings that are ordinarily shrouded by veils of culture. For some time one myth has had a particular magnetism for me—the myth of Antaeus.

According to legend, the earth (Ge) was the mother of Antaeus. Like so many of the subjects of Greek mythology, Antaeus was half god, half man. He controlled a part of North Africa by the use of his limitless strength. Whenever a stranger passed through the country, Antaeus would require the stranger to wrestle him. The stranger would always be defeated, and Antaeus would then put him to death.

These contests were not always easy, and sometimes his opponent would throw him to the earth. However, this was the source of his unbeatable strength. Each time he was thrown to the earth he was in touch with his mother, and from her he derived fresh strength. Unlike his opponents, as the match progressed Antaeus became stronger and stronger, until he was invincible.

But as powerful as he seemed, the source of his strength also held the potential for his undoing. When Hercules entered the domain of Antaeus, he was able to perceive that Antaeus' prodigious strength was renewed by contact with his mother, and acting upon this realization, he lifted Antaeus into the air, far from the support of his mother, and rendered him utterly helpless. Holding him high off the earth, Hercules was able to crush Antaeus to death.

The myth of Antaeus appealed to me as a metaphor for my own experience, for I had felt strong and able to deal with anything in life, and then I became suddenly like the helpless Antaeus, suspended in midair, no longer connected with the source of my strength: my earthly body. Antaeus was still Antaeus, and I was still me, but without supports we were both helpless, estranged from our sources of physical power. I felt as though I were cut off from the elemental functions and activities which had grounded me. I was quite literally separated from the earth, for while I spent my time in an iron lung, in a bed, or in a wheelchair, my feet almost never touched the ground.

But more important, I believe, was being separated from so many of the elemental routines that occupy people. Even if I would work, I did not have any experience of physical exertion. I could not, on my own, assume the familiar positions of standing, sitting, and lying down. I was even separated from my breathing, as it was done by a machine. I felt no longer connected with the familiar roles

I had known in family, work, sports. My place in the culture was gone.

Later, a new realization began to emerge. In many respects what happened to me was also happening to many other late-twentieth-century Americans. They too had lost their familiar grounding. Living in cities, in high-rise buildings, many people have lost all connection with the soil. They stand on concrete streets and move about effortlessly in automobiles. The connections between food, earth, and the cycles of weather are remote to the city dweller, other than as a business abstraction. Work is separated from its products, and few people have a grasp of the connections between their separate tasks and the useful effect of their work.

The liberation movements have left many people not tethered to any clear continuity in their lives. They are freed from the usual social roles in marriage and family, and are often uncertain what would provide security and satisfaction. They are even freed from some of the connections with their own biology. Birth-control pills make sexuality an option without the fear of conception, for example.

Freedom has deprived twentieth-century Americans of many familiar guideposts and pathways for moving through life. They are confronted by a bewildering array of options.

In an environment that is rapidly and continuously changing, no one's past experience is adequate. To assume that it should be is a disability. Sooner or later, we're all disabled because it's impossible to always do what we would like to do. There is a kinship between my disability's effect on me and the effect of change on abie-bodied people. We struggle individually and we struggle collectively, but we all struggle.

In a larger sense Antaeus, Oedipus, Sisyphus, and all of the heroes of Greek mythology symbolize the struggle to survive. It is our destiny in the evolutionary scheme to struggle—in that we are all alike—but each person must struggle in his own way, and seek his own meaning.

I am separated from the world by my disability and must live in exile apart from it. Yet I am also a part of the same world, and like all others, I live in a world within worlds, all related and interrelated, and each reflects the other. What I see from my point of view is also what I see in the universe.

Although I am a prisoner of my own perceptions, it is impossible for me to avoid the recognition that there is a great deal more in the universe than within me. My disability has been a wise teacher in helping me to discover some ways of realizing that. It has given me an occasional passage from my individual prison into the light of what is beyond.

When I was growing up, I learned that I must "make something of myself" and make a place in the world. Making the necessary changes to *become* something and to find a place were acts of will and effort. I learned that those things were possible if I was willing to work, to plan, to expend effort, and to struggle.

The implications were clear. I was "not enough" to begin with, and there was not a place for me in the world without my making it. Order had to be created. I had to change myself through discipline and effort. The world had to be changed to make it a better place to live in. Self-improvement was required, and the world had to be civilized. Willful, enforced change was the only kind that I learned.

My disability has taught me that there is also another kind of change. I reluctantly learned about it through defeat. I faced something that no amount of work, effort, planning, or struggle could give me. Defeated on all fronts, I had to learn how to surrender and accept what I had become, what I did not want to be.

Learning to surrender and accept what I had not chosen gave me knowledge of a new kind of change and a new kind of experience which I had not anticipated. It was a paradoxical change.

When I stopped struggling, working to change, and found means of accepting what I had already become, I discovered that that changed me. Rather than feeling disabled and inadequate as I anticipated I would, I felt whole again. I experienced a sense of well-being and a fullness which I had not known before. I felt at one not only with myself but with the universe.

This was not change that had been wrought by struggle, work, and effort, but rather by learning how not to struggle, how to give in, to stand aside and let truth emerge. It was not the tragic truth I expected at all.

When I allowed myself to face conditions that seemed intolerable and experiences that seemed unthinkable, in their reality they changed. They changed from what seemed to be horrible to something only acceptable at first, then both interesting and fulfilling.

I learned that to make a place for myself in the world, it was not always necessary to struggle, for I had a place already within me. As I became familiar with that place and increasingly trusting of it, I discovered that there was also a place for me in the world.

When I stopped trying to figure out how to get out of my predicament, and got involved with it instead, I discovered that the unpleasant and disagreeable aspects changed. As I allowed myself to be fully where and who I was in this moment, without planning for the next—this moment, this place, and I myself changed.

Sometimes the fullness I experience here and now is greater than I have ever experienced before. There is no want, no deficit, nothing larger, nothing smaller, nothing stronger, nothing weaker. There is only this alone. It is enough.

To be here and to sense the wonder, the awe, the horror, the tragedy, the comedy, is the privilege of life. I do not need to master it by changing it; nor is it my master.

So I could also be Hercules holding Antaeus in midair. I was created with the power of Hercules and the weakness of Antaeus, and both are parts of a larger me.

Feeling grounded is not so much a matter of the position of my body, or what it is in contact with, as a matter of making firm contact with whatever there is. Grounding is not a matter of touching the earth or touching the familiar or the desired alone, but can also be achieved whatever the conditions are. It can occur only, however, in the immediacy of the present moment and the immediacy of the space in which I exist.

But being who I am provides me with transcendence as well. The level of my consciousness and awareness rises, and well it should, for I am a part of an evolutionary process.

That evolution goes on everywhere, every moment in everything. When I have a glimpse of that process, I am in touch with the power of the universe, with its ever-ascending evolutionary force. So to become grounded is paradoxically also to transcend what is here and now for what is to come.

True continuity exists not in man-made plans for the future or in the memories of the past, but in riding with the continuity that is the heritage of all living things. Our momentary states allow us to move with the tides of time, and the creation and dissolution of all things.

The pulses of the universe are also the rhythms of being alive. The human expressions of those rhythms are to move out and engage the world and to retreat and assimilate. There are times for activity in the world, and times of activity within. Each requires full attention and commitment.

The rhythm must be allowed to make the choice of engaging the world or surrendering to what it has provided. The choice is best made by turning to a wisdom larger than any simple set of human beliefs. That wisdom emerges both from within and from without. It must be taken in this moment, in this place, as it appears.

I had sought a solution that I could grasp in my mind, an idea or a method that I could hold on to forever. But this blinded me to the rhythms and pulses of life in the universe. I had elevated either the struggle for mastery over events or the peacefulness of surrender to a level of a plan, but the plan was appropriate only to the conditions I had just experienced. The struggle is as meaningful as the peace. Both have the potential of turning into moments of magic and of wonder. I no longer wish to be set against myself or against the world. I wish to listen to the timeless, spaceless state that is paradoxically here and now.

12

Is It Possible to Be Disabled and Healthy at the Same Time?

In New England early in the last century, concern about the dismal state of worldly affairs led religious groups to predict that the end of the world was near. Several independent religious groups predicted that the end would come on a particular day, creating near-panic among the populace. In midday the sky unseasonably darkened and a chill wind began to blow, creating an ominous sense of gloom. The state legislature was in session, and its members were not immune from the pervasive fear that extended across the land. So it was that one of its members rose from his chair and addressed the Speaker of the Assembly: "Mr. Speaker, in view of the fact that this may be the end of the world, I move that we adjourn."

The Speaker, a distinguished elder, thoughtfully pondered the motion for a long time. Finally he spoke: "Gentlemen, it may or it may not be the end of the world. *If it is not,* we have important business to transact. If, however, *it is* the end of the world, I, for one, would wish to be at my station, doing my duty, when it comes."

FOR THREE DECADES I have been a double agent. I am both a physician and a disabled person, and I have spent large amounts of time on both sides of the health-care system. I know what the world looks like from the doctor and patient perspectives.

There are four certain simple conclusions that I have come to from my unique vantage point. First, and most obvious, the world looks very different from the standpoint of a physician and from the standpoint of a disabled person. The second is that what seems right and good from a doctor's point of view is often not the same as what seems right and good from the patient's perspective. The third point is that generally speaking, it is better to be a doctor than a patient, and not only because it is more blessed to give than to receive. And finally, if you have to be a patient, you are also better off being a doctor as well.

These simple—perhaps simplistic—conclusions have provided me with a basis for considering the question: Is it possible to be disabled and healthy at the same time?

For over thirty years I have been judged in various

circumstances, both medical and community, as "permanently disabled." That I cannot move my arms and legs, breathe on my own, seems firmly established, and will not change in this life.

What it means to be healthy and what it means to be disabled are not the same to me today as they once were.

A most benign observation has been made to me on many occasions. It is usually phrased thus: "I don't think of you as disabled." It is a strange statement, considering my physical condition.

I understand what is meant by the statement, I believe. It is intended to be a positive comment on my life—that I appear to be productive, to enjoy life, and my disability does not seem to interfere with my life in any way.

Yet from the standpoint of my medical condition, the statement is patently false. Disability is indeed a part of my reality, and a part which will not go away.

How real is the contradiction? It represents a matter of perspective, and is a matter of selective attention to different aspects of me. Each is true, but depends on a focus. The physician is committed to identifying disease and eradicating it. A side effect is that if disease is not eliminated and the person remains disabled, the case represents a failure and the physician may feel as though he has not done his job fully.

If I consider my physical disability from the physician standpoint, I am a failure, and I represent an inadequate result. Chronic patients and the crippled are awkward for the health-care system, and so many physicians prefer not to deal with these "failures." This perspective, however, is not limited to those who have M.D. degrees. It is pervasive in our society.

The preoccupation of medicine with disease and its eradication is as it should be. But this physician commitment also results in a negative attitude about anything that interferes with the recognition of illness. Physicians know from experience that avoidance of recognition may cause neglect of treatment that in turn leads to failure. So when a physician encounters a patient who denies or ignores his illness and will not accept its reality, he considers that a dangerous attitude, and one which is in itself pathological.

I am a permanently disabled patient who has the health-care or physician perspective. It's a difficult double bind. I am continuously aware of my pathology and my disability, and it once represented a failure to me as well as to those who cared for me. Moreover, patients who aren't doctors are very apt to adopt this physician perspective, since they spend so much of their time in contact with the health-care system. The effect may be disastrous.

I recall a fellow patient who was physically disabled in ways that were similar to mine. He always insisted that he would "soon be back on the golf course." The staff could see that he would never play golf again, and believed his attitude was pathological and an interference in his recovery. They confronted him forcefully with their view of "reality." He accepted the reality of his medical condition and never spoke of golf again. Unfortunately, his desire to live also came to an end. He gave up and died.

Disabled and Healthy at the Same Time? • 177

Denial of illness has been regarded negatively and as interference with good health. Indeed, for patients with acute illness that *can* be cured, early recognition and appropriate treatment is essential. But it is necessary to look deeper into the full significance of denial in order to understand its meaning for the permanently disabled who must live within their limitations.

In recent years, a series of studies of Massachusetts General Hospital have revealed a new aspect of denial of illness. Thomas Hackett and his colleagues have studied myocardial infarction patients in a coronary-care unit. They have found an apparently puzzling piece of data. It is that the psychological mechanism of denial of illness among heart attack patients is positively correlated with their survival. That is, rather than having a negative effect on the patient, denial has a positive effect, and those who deny the full significance of their illness are more apt to survive than are those who "face reality" as perceived by the physician. So far as I know, this is the first scientific study that suggests something positive about denial of illness.

This appears to be an example of two negatives making a positive. Denial and illness both have a negative connotation, but together under these conditions they seem to produce something positive, motivating patients to survive. These results then seem both illogical and contrary to the prevailing view among those in medical care.

I was fascinated by these results, and I carefully examined the data these scientists published. I noted that what they described as denial of illness could be interpreted from another point of view, one which I believe makes their results more understandable. For example, a patient who states, "It's not my heart I'm worried about, it's my wife," is one of their cases. Indeed, this may be seen as an example of denial of illness. However, from another standpoint, that of the patient's *whole* life, it may be seen as an affirmation of something he values, rather than a denial of illness.

Indeed, his wife may be more important to him than his heart, or metaphorically, she may be his heart. Focusing his attention away from his heart and onto what makes his life worth living may well be what produces his positive results, rather than the act of denial.

The patient should not be asked to choose between his physical life and his reason for living. A man who insists in the face of serious illness, "I can't be sick now, I've got three kids to send to college," may be doing himself a greater service than the man who easily accepts his illness. The health-care system, of necessity, should focus on the illness and its treatment. The patient, on the other hand, must hold out for himself the things that make life worth living.

The World Health Organization's definition of health has wisely taken into account the two perspectives we have considered. That definition includes both an absence of illness and a positive sense of well-being. These two perspectives do not occupy the same conceptual space; that is, they do not overlap, but describe different things.

If health is defined as the absence of illness, then zero, or absence, is the goal. From the zero, on a linear scale, one

Disabled and Healthy at the Same Time? · 179

could conceive of degrees of illness as -1, -2, -3, etc. This definition, however, does not attend to any attitudes or feelings which are positive.

If health is defined in terms of its positive attributes, the feeling of well-being, positive strength and attitude, then the scale is quite different. It would begin with zero and continue on the plus side; that is, there would be degrees of wellness ($+1$, $+2$, $+3$, etc.).

Under most conditions, if a person is ill, he also does not have a sense of well-being. Certainly this is the case in acute medical conditions. However, since the concepts of illness and health in a positive sense do not necessarily overlap, it opens several possibilities.

We are all familiar with the hypochondriac who has no apparent physical disease but does not have a sense of well-being at all. Instead, he continually examines himself for evidences of new illnesses which cannot be confirmed. For the person who so accepts an illness or disability that he is no longer aware of it, an almost opposite situation exists. His attention may be entirely on his sense of well-being instead.

The two different World Health Organization definitions make the apparent contradictions about disability and health possible. It would be entirely possible, thus, for a person to have both a sense of well-being and a serious illness at the same time.

The word "health" is derived from the Greek root word "holos." That root has given rise to several related words: whole, heal, hale, holy, holistic. Holos refers then to positive states of health, to wholeness and to the transcendent holy.

The "dis-," as in "disability," is taken to mean apart or away from, and is derived from "di"—meaning twice. Disabled, then, refers to a person who is apart from being able, or who, rather than being whole, is divided in two parts. Disease apart from ease has a similar derivation.

If we scrutinize a person selectively to discover his weaknesses, his faults, or the ways in which he is deficient, we can always find some, although certainly this may vary in degree or obviousness. If, on the other hand, we look to the ways in which that same person is whole or healthy, we may also be able to discover many things. So it will appear that the point of reference will determine which of the characteristics we will find. "Seek and ye shall find." The choice between these perspectives has already been considered.

We human beings cannot grasp the totality of reality. We are limited by what it is that draws our attention. We habitually look for those things we expect to find and view the world selectively. Our view is therefore slightly warped. But habits are alterable, and new ones can be acquired by practice.

For example, during frequent moments of special candor and intimacy between my patients and me, I have often been asked, "How do you stand not being able to move?" Although I am appreciative of the openness which leads to the question, it often surprises me, because I am totally unaware of being disabled at the time. To answer requires a

Disabled and Healthy at the Same Time? · 181

shift in my positive attention from what I am involved in (my experience of closeness with this patient) to thinking about those things which I am unable to do. The shift is from feeling able and healthy to feeling disabled and sick.

It is far more practical to consider a somewhat different way of understanding the meaning of health and disability. When a person sees those aspects of the world that are affirmative, those things he can do that are of value, he experiences a state of health. When, on the other hand, he views the world from the standpoint of what he cannot do, he is disabled regardless of his physical condition. The experiencing of health or disability is a momentary phenomenon, which depends on a frame of reference and a selectivity of attention.

From the standpoint of my disability, much of my life could be said to represent an implied denial of illness, but from another point of view it is a striving to develop what is available to me and what I can value.

The experience of wholeness, of necessity, is in the here and now. When one attends to those things not in the here and now, he is more likely to divide himself by his struggle with the past or with the future. It is possible, as the psychologist Gordon Allport has said, "to be wholehearted and half right at the same time"; and, emphasizing the essentialness of the here and now, Kierkegaard observed: "Purity of heart is to will one thing"—one thing at a time.

The problem is in getting stuck in choosing one map instead of the whole territory. The territory must continually be traversed, and is open to movement. The map is man-made and static. We need both a guide and the reality to touch. We must guard against the guide becoming a Procrustean bed of disability. To shut out the changing flow of life is to accept one man's wisdom above the wisdom of the universe.

To live in the here and now is not the same as living *for* the here and now. Each of us needs to find a purpose as well. One choice always leaves another unchosen. In going toward one, another is left behind, and we are what we become in the quest we have set for ourselves.

But health is not only an individual experience; it encompasses relationships with others as well. To have a sense of wholeness and well-being requires human connections for nourishment. I have been fortunate to have had support from family and friends even though I have not infrequently felt deprived. Increasingly I realize that when that happens it is because I am not open to the form in which the support is offered, preferring instead to insist that it be in accordance with my expectations.

My relationship with Rita has been central to my personal sense of health and well-being.

Together, we have traveled widely in the United States and Europe. We have had experiences that would be rewarding to any able-bodied persons. We have done interesting things and met interesting people. We have made good friends and very few enemies.

My energy and physical strength have, as is to be expected, slowly but inexorably declined. My workday has shortened consistent with reduced breathing capacity and

Disabled and Healthy at the Same Time? · 183

sitting tolerance. Each functional loss is painful, and I am never prepared for it—although I anticipate it. But I am learning, and doing it a little better. Although I experience the denial, bargaining, rage, and sadness of grief with each stage of decline, it becomes smoother and more graceful too. How I feel is well expressed by something William James once said. He had lived a long life, and was asked if he believed in life after death. His answer was: "Never much so, but more as I grow older, because I am just becoming fit to live."

Rita and I have now been married nearly thirty-five years. In that time we have always been facing some "minor inconvenience" or "major problem." These problems, whatever their size, have not kept us from the more important business of living.

An exception for us to the "normal" pattern of married life has been that we have had no children, although we vigorously engaged in all of the activities and procedures that ordinarily would have produced them. My concerns about my survival, my ability to support a family, and my ability to engage in parental activities created some ambivalence on my part. Rita's desire, however, was straightforward, and so we involved ourselves in creating the required context for children with enthusiasm and pleasure. Still, the results were disappointing. I have learned nothing if not that nature is full of surprises.

Several years ago, the ultimate irony of ironies occurred. Rita developed a disabling rheumatoid arthritis. This was no minor inconvenience, for Rita was a person who had always expressed herself physically with grace, strength, and skill. It meant no more tennis for her, no more vigorous gardening, and no more building projects of the sort she had always enjoyed. Her major mode of orientation to the world was interrupted.

And most of all, it required reorientation in how we lived together.

Rita's physical capabilities had to do for both of us, and had been the very basis of our living together like any other married couple. She provided most of my considerable physical care when we first married, so we had to learn to live together in the most intimately demanding of circumstances. Now we had to live with an entire staff of employees to help us with the activities of everyday life. It was especially intrusive and painful for Rita, who had always been used to doing things for herself.

Our household now includes many others who help with my care and other personal functions. For both of us, struggles between personal autonomy and dependence moved to a new and more destabilizing plane.

However, this process was not without rewards, for the intimacy that we have had between us has now been extended to include others. Each of those we employed became a part of our lives, bringing their own unique needs and varying perspectives on the world. They were frequently very different from the views that Rita and I share, so we had to learn to live with many personal differences, and to respect them. We have not been spared the trials of having adolescents in the household, even though we did not give birth to them ourselves.

Most of those who have come to help have been young people, students and others in transition. The length of time during which they remain in the household is usually no more than a couple of years. This creates further problems of destabilization, and we are constantly in the process of training and retraining helpers.

But there is a more important aspect of the enlarged household. Although we now say we did not have children of our own, we can add that "other people did that for us." Indeed, our home has become a second family for nearly all who have come to help us. We have not replaced their natural parents, but as one of our helpers once said, "You have refined what my parents began."

Our "finishing school" has had its share of personal dilemmas, drug and sexual problems. It has produced body builders, journalists, engineers, surfers, physicians, psychologists, businessmen, and many others.

They have taught us more than we have taught them. They have given us more than we have given them. They have expanded our understanding of the meaning of relationship and love, and they have taught us more again about the meanings of kinship and kindness. They became the intermediate connections between our intimacy and our relationship to all people.

It is not easy to know what we should call these helpers/teachers/friends/children/students, but we know that we never forget them, and it appears that they never forget us. We attend their weddings, christenings, graduations, and other symbols of growth. When they have gone out into the world, they continue to call, write, and return regularly for visits and vacations, often with spouses and children attached.

If someone were to ask if I would like to return to being able-bodied, my first question would be: "What would I have to give up?" If someone were to ask Rita and me if we would like to return to her pre-rheumatoid arthritis situation, our first question would also be: "What would we have to give up?" We have received some disguised gifts from each of these traumatic events. I do not minimize their very traumatic nature. Things happened that we did not want, that we fought against to keep from happening, things that were painful and disruptive. But they brought unexpected opportunities once they happened, and there was no way of turning back. In order to see the opportunities, though, you must accept what happened as if you have chosen it. Whatever comes next, I hope I will be able to remember that lesson.

Both my inner world and the outer world are in continuous change, and do not always move at the same pace. How I position myself, my world, in relationship to the outer world is critical to how I feel.

When I became disabled, I could no longer derive support from familiar positions. I have found, however, that it is possible to derive support from whatever the immediate opportunities may be. So long as I am open to the messages of my inner world and I allow contact with the outside world to be clear and firm, I feel supported. My senses, my sight, hearing, touch, smell, taste, and sense of position, are my points of contact. They are supports that are always present if I will admit them to my awareness.

But my reach must exceed my grasp. How I live here and now is determined by what I seek. What I live *for* and the frame of reference that creates determine what I find. I must have a reason for getting up in the morning, for doing what I am doing. I must be going someplace. A firm hold on this moment and this space is not enough.

The horizons I look for may change. They are represented by a series of almost trivial but intermediate purposes: my wife's return, a visit with my mother, the dinner I anticipate, the friends who will visit, the next patient that I will see, this book that I am writing.

But what are these trivial purposes for? What is it that I seek beyond these benchmarks? Often I am uncertain, but sometimes it becomes clear.

Since I can see elements of truth in all religions and philosophies—and no one seems sufficient in itself—I am not continuously guided by some relatively simple frame of reference. The future that I move toward has only sketchy details for me. It is a future which I cannot fully comprehend, but which faith tells me exists, and which is worthwhile.

It is not a future which is limited to my own destiny in my body and in my time, but something much larger. My inner world revolves around some mysterious something which I call "me." The whole universe revolves around something even more mysterious and awesome. But there are times, increasingly more frequent and of longer duration, when I and that larger something are in synchrony. Those are the times when boundaries disappear, when time disappears and space is without meaning. At these moments all conventional terms pale in their attempts to describe what there is, for it is beyond peace, beyond joy, beyond tragedy, beyond comedy, and well beyond health and disability.

ABOUT THE AUTHOR

ARNOLD BEISSER is a graduate of Stanford University and its medical school. He is Clinical Professor of Psychiatry at UCLA, a Life Fellow of the American Psychiatric Association, and a recipient of its Gold Achievement Award. He has published over 100 articles, reviews, book chapters, and books, including *Madness in Sports* and *Mental Health Consultation*.